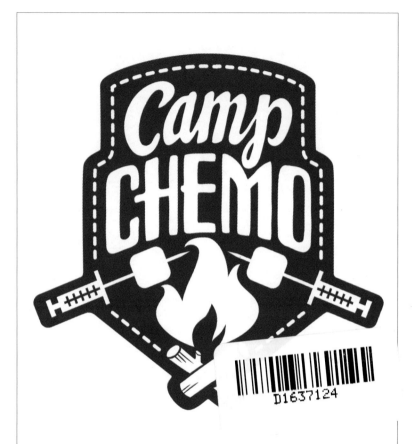

Postcards home from
metastatic breast cancer

Camille Scheel

Camp Chemo

ISBN 13: 978-1-59298-850-1

Library of Congress Catalog Number: 2015947964

Printed in the United States of America

First Printing: 2015

19 18 17 16 15   5 4 3 2 1

Edited by Peter Clowney and Wendy Weckworth.

Cover and interior design by Laura Drew.
Cover illustration © Kevin Cannon.

Beaver's Pond Press
7108 Ohms Lane
Edina, MN 55439–2129
952-829-8818
www.beaverspondpress.com

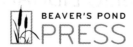

DEDICATED TO THOSE LIVING WITH CANCER
AND TO THOSE WHOSE HEALING FROM CANCER
IS COMPLETED BY PASSAGE FROM THIS WORLD.

For Wade,
my best reader, partner, and friend.

ᕲ

For Vivian and Jackson,
you continue to make the world a better place
by your very presence in it.

Introduction

On Friday, September 14, 2007, I was diagnosed with Stage III lobular carcinoma—breast cancer. I was thirty-eight.

The story that follows is a real-time blog on CaringBridge.org, a nonprofit online resource where patients and their families can create a personal website to share medical news with family and friends. The blog stemmed from my immediate need to communicate about my prognosis and experiences with my family and friends.

My body no longer felt like home. These "postcards" were written as blog posts to my new home, my CaringBridge community of family, friends, neighbors, and coworkers. Wade, my husband, made the first CaringBridge entries.

My daughter, Vivian, was six at the time of my diagnosis, and my son, Jackson, was one.

All doctors and other patients are referred to with pseudonyms and any identifying details are obscured. Our cats, Rocko (a.k.a. Dr. Rocko), Cedric, and Shu Shu, and dogs, Savannah and Lupita, consented to the use of their real names.

This book isn't intended to diagnose, treat, cure, or prevent any disease. However, it is to help you understand one life with cancer, and perhaps, by extension, open you to insights about your own life, with or without cancer.

stage III
New Kid at Camp

A New Website

Tuesday, September 25, 2007, 9:36 p.m.

Hey, everybody,

Wade (the husband) here to give a very abbreviated update. Camille is doing great. There were some setbacks, but they were manageable, and well . . . we managed them. I'm happy to say Camille's breast surgeon, Dr. Farah, told us he "got it all." The margins from the lumpectomy were clear in the final pathology report, indicating that he was able to remove all the "visible" cancer. Camille is doing great, but her struggles aren't over; we still get to look forward to four months of chemotherapy, then radiation, and then additional medication to give those little cancer f!$*%s the final one-two punch. Thank you soooo much for all your support over the last couple of days. The calls, the flowers, the privacy—and especially thanks for the prayers, karma, and the positive thinking. We will definitely have to have a survivor party sometime in the late winter or early spring.

Love to you all,
Wade

PET Scan

Wednesday, September 26, 2007, 2:57 p.m.

Hi to all again, it's Wade.

Camille is in the PET scan machine as I write. We'll be picking her up from the hospital in just a few hours, and as you can imagine, the kids can't wait to see her.

For those of you who know the strong personality that is Vivian, you can probably imagine that this has been quite hard on her. Please include her in your prayers for strength and understanding.

Camille will begin updating this blog soon, and you should all know that for her to stay in bed for almost three days was the real torture. (Ain't she grand?) She's anxious to get back to work and giving us orders around the house.

Thanks for the encouragement,
Wade

Stage III

Wednesday, September 26, 2007, 8:49 p.m.

I'm home from the hospital! While I'm totally exhausted, it's great to be home. Being free of needles for at least a few days is such a happy prospect. Family was visiting tonight, but now the kids are asleep, and I'll be sleeping soon too. Poor Wade is cleaning the kitchen before he goes to bed.

The PET scan confirmed no more cancer! The diagnosis is officially Stage III, which means it traveled from my breast to my lymph nodes. The surgeon removed eleven nodes, and six were found to have cancer.

If you visit, two things to keep in mind: we're not saying "cancer" to Vivian. She knows I had surgery to remove something that was growing wrong. She knows I'll need medicine, but we haven't discussed that my hair will fall out. She's only six, so we don't want to scare her. Also, if you visit, do try to pay some attention to Vivian—she's been such a big girl about everything. Already her little Swedish stiff upper lip is showing. She says that everything is fine, even when you can see the concern in her little eyes.

Jackson doesn't know what's going on. In some ways, I hate having to deal with this when he's only one year old, but I'm glad he won't remember any of it. It's hard to believe he was still nursing just a few weeks ago when I found the lump. When I found out I'd have to stop nursing him immediately, I cried for hours. It was such a shock—I hadn't realized nursing would have to stop after the breast MRI that was required before surgery. How do you tell a baby he needs to end, immediately, that special activity he's loved his whole life? It was difficult, but I knew it was best for his health and mine.

Luckily, both kids have been cared for by my mom several days per week since they were babies. Her calming presence is helping keep life as normal as possible for them now. She's a retired nurse, so even when I was a kid, she took great care of me whenever I was sick. Her expert care of me continues today, and I'm glad the kids are also benefiting from having a wonderful grandma.

The last few days have been an emotional roller coaster. From the high highs of receiving the "no more surgery" news to the low lows of "wow, I have cancer—is there something I could have done to prevent this?"

I have two to three weeks to heal from the surgery. During that time, I'll have more tests, including a heart scan, to make sure I'm healthy enough for chemo. Before my hair falls out, I hope to meet with my hairdresser to discuss a short haircut. Then I'll donate my hair to the charity Locks of Love, which makes wigs for kids experiencing permanent medical hair loss. The American Cancer Society has a whole packet on beauty during chemo, and I look forward to experimenting with some new looks.

Chemo will last four months. It's a bummer, but it's hard to get too upset about a treatment that will save my life, even if it sucks in the short term.

Thank you for your love and support!
Camille

Back to the Office

Friday, September 28, 2007, 9:15 p.m.

Today, I went into the office for two hours, and it was so great to be back at work. My manager, Barb, provided some sound advice: ease back. Don't rush it. But I long to be back for real. It was nice to see my dear colleagues again. They're so very supportive.

Feeling good about work is starting to ease my financial worries connected to this disease. Despite having "good" health insurance, we'll still have to fork over a ton of cash for my "maximum out-of-pocket expense." Hopefully, the loss of wages from my surgical recovery will be minimized if I can keep up a good pace when I'm at the office. Even though I work at a nonprofit, most of my compensation is commission, so as long as I work hard, my paychecks will keep up.

Physically, I'm feeling good, but I tire very quickly. Two long naps kept me going strong today.

The one current source of pain is the drainage tube (yes, it's as gross as it sounds). It's a one-centimeter-wide tube with two bulbs attached. One bulb is under my skin; the other is at the end of the tube. A few times a day, we need to empty the pouch and measure the amount of fluid so we can report to the doctor if there's too much. I'm looking forward to my next doctor's appointment when the gross drainage tube will be removed.

My sense of gratitude grows daily with all the kind words, flowers, cookies, meals, and offers of help that keep coming in. Still, our greatest need is for continued prayer and positive thoughts. If your place of worship has a prayer list, please add me to it. My belief in the power of prayer grows daily.

We still haven't said the *C* word to Vivian, and she hasn't been asking any questions about my health since I returned home from the hospital. Her fantastic school social worker had a talk with Vivian, who seems to be doing well, according to her. Jackson had a few difficult nights after the speed weaning, but now he's getting back to his easygoing self. Both kids are getting more cookies than ever before!

Thunderstorm Beauty
Sunday, September 30, 2007, 8:45 p.m.

Woke up this morning to a beautiful thunderstorm. No pain at all upon waking! No nightmares last night. Plus, I only woke once to take medication. What a great night.

The good night was followed by a good morning at church. The sermon was on envy. It's strange, but in many ways I envy myself—the me I was a month ago. I envy my freedom from pain and fear. I envy my petty worries from last month.

Before dinner, I went to the gym to walk and ride the bike. Not a very vigorous workout, but I wanted to at least go there to get past that first time back.

Overall, a good day.

Camp Chemo
Monday, October 1, 2007, 9:48 p.m.

Went to work. It was good to see people and get a few things done. Concentration is much more difficult than before the diagnosis. This afternoon, Dr. Farah removed my drainage tube. I couldn't believe when I saw the big bulb that had been under my skin for a full week—no wonder it hurt! Now that the main source of pain has been removed, I'm noticing all the smaller aches and pains leftover from surgery.

Next week, I start physical therapy to learn how to prevent lymphedema, a complication that can arise due to the removal of eleven lymph nodes from my right armpit. Lymphedema causes painful swelling and hardening of the tissue between the skin to the bone due to backed-up lymph fluid. It can cause serious infections if left untreated. The therapists will teach me some preventative exercises. I've already learned some ways to prevent it—no blood draws or blood pressures taken on my right arm, for example. Only an electric razor should be used to shave my right armpit. I have to be careful to avoid burns, including sunburns, on my right arm. I should carry my purse, briefcase, and so on over my left arm. I'm also not allowed to get bug bites on my right arm. Lymphedema can appear as many as five years into the future, so these changes need to become habits. The main point of the physical therapy, though, is to regain my range of motion—my arm doesn't move as far up or over as it did before the lumpectomy.

Chemo will start in two or three weeks. Before I begin, Wade and I will attend a chemo class that I've been jokingly calling Camp Chemo. I'm considering getting some Camp Chemo T-shirts printed up ahead of time for myself and the other participants, but they might not find it so funny. I keep imagining Camp Chemo will include songs around the campfire, roasting marshmallows, and telling ghost stories. Probably not the case, but I'll keep you posted.

I have the green light to call my oncologist and set my first appointment. Before the chemo starts, my heart will be tested to make sure it's strong enough for the chemo, which can cause heart damage.

Sinking In
Wednesday, October 3, 2007, 5:16 a.m.

The flowers people sent are dying, the Vicodin is running out, and it's all starting to sink in. This must be what it's like after a spouse's funeral when the guests leave, the food runs out, and the surviving spouse starts to feel alone. Cards still come in the mail, and I still get lots of phone calls, but the initial shock is wearing off. Shock was my friend because when things were moving so fast, I didn't have time to panic. Not that I'm panicking now, but yikes, every time I pick up my purse with my left hand instead of my right, I remember, *Oh* yes, I have cancer in my lymph nodes.

The bugaboo with cancer is there isn't one set course of treatment. My surgeon described a whole cookbook of drugs and treatments my oncologist will consider for me. Ironic, because I will be literally cooked during the radiation process.

I'm a planner, but there's no way to know if I'll just feel sick for two days after each treatment but still be able to work or if I'll be knocked on my butt for a whole week. That uncertainty drives me crazy.

Yesterday, I attended my first cancer support group. Maybe it was a bad idea, because it scared me. The women in the group talked about nausea, burns during radiation, and worse. One woman got lymphedema and has to wear a compression garment on her arm for the rest of her life. Talk about a fashion faux pas. Most of them are retirement age and had grown children before they were diagnosed with cancer, so they couldn't answer my questions about working and parenting during treatment.

Here's the downside of being in sales and paid by commission: I don't get paid if I don't work. The current unknowns are frightening because I still want to be at the top of my professional game. I read in my National Institutes of Cancer booklet that cancer patients are protected under the Americans with Disabilities Act, which means I can't be fired for having cancer. However, that doesn't do much good when you're only paid for your sales success. Normally, I thrive on the challenge of commission. Right now, I long for a good, old-fashioned salary. Wade is a potter and has a pottery day job where he works piece rate, so he's paid for his actual output. Plus, he's at the start of the production line, so if he doesn't get his work done, many other people (and their families) suffer by not having enough work to do a few days down the line. Needless to say, we're both feeling a ton of pressure to keep working through all of this.

I could feel the power of your prayers when I was in the hospital. Maybe I should start praying again also. You'd think I'd be praying all the time now, but the distraction of work and the joy of getting that disgusting drainage tube removed have rendered me too exhausted to think about much else. Maybe I'll start napping again. I miss the naps.

Uncertainty Reduction

Wednesday, October 3, 2007, 8:16 p.m.

Today started out with the glass half-empty. Not a natural state for me. Every little worry that has crossed my mind in the past two weeks came to the forefront this morning.

The biggest was waiting for another two and a half weeks for the first meeting with the oncologist. So I called this afternoon to see if I could get in sooner, and he said to come by at eight tomorrow morning. File that under "be careful what you wish for." The treatment won't start any earlier, but this way I can educate myself on what to expect.

During my master's program in interpersonal communication, I learned about uncertainty reduction theory. The basic principle: people don't like to face the unknown. In interpersonal communication, this is evident when strangers ask questions of each other to find common ground. Another example is that much of human communication is actually scripted before it happens. Don't believe me? Ask ten people tomorrow, "How are you?" and I guarantee that nine will reply, "Fine." Because that's the script. You probably have different scripts with different people, but it's all because leaving too much up in the air drives us human beings bananas.

So according to uncertainty reduction theory, I can rest easy tonight, knowing that I'll be able to reduce my angst tomorrow morning by eliminating some of those pesky unknowns. Hopefully, I won't get another scoopful of "be careful of what you wish for."

Chemotherapy Details

Thursday, October 4, 2007, 6:25 p.m.

Dr. Anderson is wonderful. His voice is calming without being condescending, and like my dear breast surgeon, Dr. Farah, Dr. Anderson has delicate hands that look very soft. Soft hands seem like a positive attribute for a doctor. Wade likes him too.

The follow-up appointment with Dr. Farah was also today. He said the healing looks great and was impressed by how high I can lift my arm. I told him I need lots of information to plan the upcoming months, and he said I'm longing for that because the cancer had stolen so much of my ability to control my life. He said I'm just trying to get some control back. I told him that I like to move at a fast pace at work and home, so my recent slowdown is really upsetting and that I want to be back at work at full capacity. He said, "You want your life to be normal again. And it's not going to be. This is like setting the reset button; everything has to change." I know he's right, but that's a tough pill to swallow.

Chemo starts on October 22. Prior to that, I have about twelve hours of doctor appointments, not even counting Camp Chemo or wig shopping. The therapy Dr. Anderson has selected is called TAC and is the most aggressive chemotherapy on the market today. It's Taxotere, Adriamycin, and Cytoxan. All will be administered intravenously. Before and after each chemo, I'll have to take handfuls of pills, including steroids. Treatment will be once every three weeks for six cycles. Nobody can say how sick I'll feel, but Dr. Farah said I'll become anemic, so I'll be very tired.

At the office today, I spoke with my bosses and now have a much brighter outlook on how to survive a slowdown at work. We'll have a strategy session next week to figure out how my colleagues can pitch in if I need help. We'll also discuss ways to maximize my time when I'm in the office. I prefer to meet with clients face-to-face, but I can be more efficient by working via e-mail and phone appointments. Plus, this will help protect my chemo-weakened immune system.

On the financial front, being entrepreneurs, Wade and I have come up with a plan to offset the medical bills. We're planning a special sale of Wade's pottery and paintings. We may also sell Camp Chemo T-shirts! It will be a chance to raise money and commune with all of you who are supporting us through our journey. Details to come!

I've realized that as long as the train is moving (doctor appointments, checking tasks off my list, and treatment), I'm pretty optimistic. Once the train stops, I start to worry. Worry can be a good thing—if it leads to action. In the past twenty-four hours, I've been able to take action on many fronts, and I've started planning to improve my situation.

Highs and Lows
Monday, October 8, 2007, 7:47 a.m.

What a roller-coaster weekend. Highs included visits from friends and family. Seeing Vivian on Sunday morning dressed in her church choir robe is like looking at a beautiful little angel. Two long walks listening to my new favorite podcast also lifted my mood.

Lows included crying all through church—the most tears I've shed AD (after diagnosis). Everything is starting to hit me at once. Luckily, a dear friend was sitting next to me and provided comfort. My surgeon told me there would be a grieving process. Now I understand.

The nightmares are back—I'm looking for something I can't find. Or I'm hiding, sometimes with Jackson. I'm not sure what I'm hiding from, but I think the nightmares could be about searching for the control I've lost over my life. Plus, I'm trying to hide myself and the kids from the consequences of how our lives are changing. My dreams have always been very transparent.

Not only is today Monday, but it's raining, so that stupid song "Rainy Days and Mondays" by the Carpenters is stuck in my head. Oh shoot, now it's stuck in your head too. Sorry about that. This is despite the extra loud volume of *The Magic School Bus* video in the background at my house right now.

This morning, after going to work for a few hours, I'll leave for my first physical therapy appointment. The range of motion in my right arm has declined in the last few days; it's sore too, like a bad case of tennis elbow. Hopefully, they'll give me exercises that will provide relief. Then I'll go back to work for the afternoon. Despite the rain and that stupid Carpenters song, it's setting up to be a good day. I can feel it.

Explaining Chemo to a Six-Year-Old
Monday, October 8, 2007, 10:41 p.m.

The physical therapist said that my range of motion should be totally back within six appointments. When she asked me to move each arm straight in front of me, as high as possible, I could move my left arm above my head, like a student ready to answer a question. My right arm got stuck in a "Heil, Hitler" position. Looking forward to that situation resolving soon.

If you're a boy, skip to the next paragraph. The other good part about today is I finally wore a normal bra again. After surgery, Dr. Farah explained that wearing a sports bra "minimizes jiggling." Once I returned to work, this presented a number of fashion challenges—very few office-appropriate tops look good with a sports bra underneath. In other girl news, my physical therapist told me that Kegels aren't enough to maintain healthy vaginal muscle tone. She recently learned a critical exercise at a conference, which involves sitting in a chair and rotating the knees forty-five degrees while activating the pelvic floor. She explained that this exercise "minimizes dribbling." So with the jiggling and dribbling minimized, I hope to feel like a (somewhat) normal woman once more.

Despite getting some new molars, Jackson is his typical happy-guy self. Vivian is having a good school year so far, and her teacher is fantastic. Her teacher did tell us Vivian has been more quiet than usual. At home, she's been showing small signs of stress, like taking longer to fall asleep at night and sticking closer to me than normal.

Wade and I have fretted from day one about how to tell her the full news about cancer. At first, I just told her something was growing wrong in my breast, so surgery would remove it. Then we started looking for children's books to introduce the word *cancer*. Many involved bald moms, crying children, children's friends making fun of the bald moms—yikes.

We recently switched to Yoplait yogurt, and I told Vivian to lick the lid and put it in a bowl so we can bring them to church for a parishioner who mails them in to Yoplait. So Vivian asked Wade, "Does the church get money from the lids?" And he replied, "No, the money goes for breast cancer research." To which she responded, "Like Mommy has?" Wow, so much for having to explain that I have cancer.

We still had to explain chemo. We told her at dinner that I need some medicine, even though the surgery was a success. I told Vivian that some side effects are really serious—like when I get tired, I'll have to sleep a lot, and sometimes she'll have to be really quiet around the house. Then I said some side effects are really silly, like my hair will come out! So I'll be bald like Daddy! She thought that was hilarious. I'm so thankful that Wade shaves his head so we could use this as an example. I explained that I'll get some wigs, maybe one that looks like the long brunette hair I have now and maybe one that looks like her blonde hair—that gave her a good laugh. I also said I might choose a pink or purple wig too. She suggested one with bangs would be cute. I told her maybe she could help me pick one, which she's excited to do. I told her that I'll need to wear a wig to stay warm when I go outside, but she and Jackson will need to get used to seeing me without hair around the house. Then she asked, "What are some of the other silly side effects of this medicine?" When I said my eyebrows and eyelashes might fall out too, she suggested I locate some false eyelashes before that happens. Girl after my own heart! She didn't seem traumatized by any of it; I wonder if she'll remain calm about it as time goes on. Talk about building character at a young age.

Loews Miami Beach

Thursday, October 11, 2007, 9:57 p.m.

Today felt like a science fiction movie. I went to the hospital and proceeded to the nuclear medicine department for my heart scan to make sure I'm fit for chemo. (I'm no stranger to nuclear medicine; I swallowed radioactive iodine a few years ago to kill my thyroid. But that's another story.) A nurse took a vial of blood and then directed me to the waiting room. She promised she'd be back in twenty-five minutes.

Sitting there, I saw a woman about my age being handed a barium "cocktail." "You seem too young to be here," I said. Turns out she's only thirty-three, with three children, the youngest in neonatal intensive care unit at the children's hospital. Her baby was born at twenty-eight weeks, weighing just two pounds. The child will be home sometime next month. The woman told me she was there taking the barium for her Crohn's disease. When I mentioned that I'd recently had barium for a CT scan, she asked, "Did they give you a straw?" Why no, they didn't. She explained that a straw helps if you put it in the back of your throat and slurp quickly; you don't taste the nasty stuff as much. Hey, you learn something new every day.

The woman told me about the severe challenges of Crohn's disease. I felt a touch of envy when she said, "It's not something that will kill me . . . ." My doctors haven't been willing to say that about cancer.

Early on, I somehow didn't think that it was possible this cancer could kill me. Now every time I have a doctor's appointment, I'm reminded this is serious stuff. A woman in her fifties walked into the waiting room, an oxygen tank trailing behind her. "What are you in for?" I asked, but the prison humor did nothing for her. Lung-cancer surgery, she said, took 25 percent of her lung and put her into a coma for a week. "I guess that's what I get for smoking," she said. Her doctor also recommended chemo, but she believes he prescribed it only because of the money he'll get. Yikes.

When the nurse finally returned for me, I went back to the nuclear medicine suite. She removed my vial of blood from a thick ceramic container and then injected it back into my arm. While I'd been chatting in the lobby with my fellow sickos, my blood had been steeping in radioactive liquid. Yum. As the nurse worked, I commented on her plastic ring with a small piece of paper in the middle. The ring looked like a miniature hospital bracelet. She told me it contained film that's constantly registering her radiation exposure. Did it ever get too high? Only once, she said, when she was working as a pharmacy intern. Interns get the crappy jobs everywhere.

After taking the heart scans, I was set free to go to physical therapy right across the street. As I walked, an amazing thought came into my head: I could run away right now. I could blow off physical therapy, drive to the airport, buy a plane ticket, and be at the Loews Miami Beach Hotel by dinnertime. I could forget that the last four weeks ever happened. I considered it all the way to physical therapy. Once at PT, I learned the restrictions I'll have with my right arm aren't for just the next five years but for the rest of my life. It's a wonder I'm not at the Lowes already.

Last night, I dreamed some family members who've known me since I was born orchestrated a major betrayal. They had conspired to stop acting like my family—instead, they wanted to kill me. I was desperately trying to escape from them and trying to protect my kids from them. Gee, what could this dream possibly be about? Maybe my body, which I've had since I was born, has now betrayed me. How much do I wish I could escape the cancer and protect my children from all the stress this is causing?

In real life, if I ever go missing, check the Loews in South Beach.

One Month
Sunday, October 14, 2007, 9:10 p.m.

Today marks one month since receiving my diagnosis. Wade and I feel like it's been two years. So many ups and downs, so much stress, so much happening it feels like time is slowing down.

Last night was a terrible night. I woke up around 1:00 a.m., worries swirling through my mind. Today was a good day for the most part, though. When people ask, "How are you?" I just say, "I'm doing fine right now," because sometimes my feelings change from moment to moment.

The worst things I worry about now are: getting the IV port installed (which happens tomorrow, and I'm dreading it); chemotherapy; lymphedema; and radiation. Even though I'm getting the best care possible, I'm already afraid of the cancer coming back.

During tornado season in Minnesota, when news crews visit sites where a home has been destroyed, the same scene always plays out. The videographer shows the damage, the flattened home and downed trees. During the interview, the homeowner appears stoic and finds a way to say, "It could have been worse. At least nobody was hurt." And I keep thinking about that—yes, it could have been worse, it could have been

Stage IV, instead of Stage III. As cancer staging goes, there is no Stage V, so at least I still have a shot at living.

Yesterday, with Wade along, I tried on wigs for the first time. It wasn't as much fun as I'd thought it would be. Both Wade and the saleswoman think that after my hair is cut (sometime this week?) it will be easier to tell how the wigs will look on me. With so much long hair, the wigs don't sit quite right. Plus, there's something about buying a wig during Halloween season that makes it seem all the more comical and weird. Looking at wigs made me sad to lose my hair, which is something I wasn't too worried about at the start. Still, hair is a small price to pay. It could have been worse.

This morning as I got ready for church, I realized that despite the many things I can't do, at least I can wear makeup and perfume. If those were restricted, I'd be in really big trouble. Even when I feel terrible, a fresh coat of makeup sure brings me back to life.

All the love and support I've been receiving daily has made such a difference. I have my own little cheering section. You're helping me heal, and for that I am so grateful. I'll continue to keep you updated with these CaringBridge posts. Or better yet, let's think of them as "postcards" from Camp Chemo.

Port Installation

Monday, October 15, 2007, 9:00 p.m.

The IV port was successfully installed today. It's a device the diameter of a quarter coin that allows the nurses to insert the chemo needle through the port instead of searching for a vein each chemo round. Even precancer, I had crappy little veins. It's a weird thing to know about yourself, but phlebotomists always complain about my tiny veins. The port is also helpful because chemo can cause the veins to collapse, making it even harder to insert a needle into already tiny veins.

The only downside of the port is that it makes scar number five. One for each of the two tumors, another for the lymph nodes, a small one for the drainage tube, and now this one. Even with lower-cut shirts, my first four won't show, but the port scar is up pretty high, so it will be obvious. I'm trying to think of these new additions to my body as battle wounds or beauty marks.

The port installation itself wasn't bad at all. In fact, I enjoyed chatting with the nurses and my cocktail waitresses (as the anesthesia nurses call themselves). They actually helped me finally understand something. Ever since I was a teenager, I've often received what seems like an odd compliment—"You have beautiful skin." I'd never think to compliment someone's skin. Today, when I met the port installation nurse, the first thing she said was, "You have beautiful skin!" I told her it's always been funny to get that compliment because when I look in the mirror I don't see it. I just see . . . me, my skin, and every little imperfection. Today, though, I went to the bathroom to put on the blue surgery hat (thank God surgery blue is my color). When I looked in the mirror, my skin really did look beautiful. I didn't see myself the way I usually do. I didn't see the imperfections. Maybe the compliment finally stuck—or maybe I'm just seeing things as they really are now. Somehow in the midst of all this ugliness, I was able to see beauty in myself that others have seen for years. What a surprising gift.

Itchy Day
Tuesday, October 16, 2007, 10:45 p.m.

I made it to work. My port is pretty painful today, and tonight it's itching like crazy. Instead of stitches, they closed the incision with glue—it looks like plastic wrap on my skin. The surgical pain makes for a bad combination of wanting to itch it but having intense pain if I touch it. Further proof that the gods are really mad at me.

On the bright side, the kids are doing great. If I can brag for a moment, Jackson is having a language explosion, and he's as polite as can be. Give him some water, milk, or a toy, and he'll say "doh, doo" (translation: thank you). He also says "bubble mower" and "more bubbles" when talking about his favorite toy. Vivian is in the accelerated math class, which she loves. She also enjoys gymnastics class and playdates with friends. I love helping with her homework; it's so cute that she has homework in first grade. I'm glad that even when I'm not feeling well I'm still able to help with her homework and reading.

Here's to an easier, less itchy day tomorrow.

The Middle of the Night
Thursday, October 18, 2007, 2:46 a.m.

If you're wondering why I'm writing in the middle of the night, it's because I have this new weird sleep pattern. By the time I lie down with Vivian to read to her at 8:00 p.m., I'm so exhausted that I fall asleep with her. Then around midnight, I move into my own bed. Then Jackson wakes around 1:00 a.m. Wade or I get up with him, and then I'm up for a little while and back to sleep around 4:00 a.m. The upside is that I get some alone time in the middle of the night. Probably good for me to have a little time all by myself to process living with cancer.

Today is the big day! Camp Chemo has arrived! Considering what a planner I normally am, I'm shocked that I've done almost no research on chemo. During the past month, I've concluded the Internet is worthless for serious, in-depth medical information. I have one book on breast cancer, and the chapter on chemo is informative but quite general. Part of me doesn't want to know all the details.

I realized that, starting with the biopsy on September 12, I've been in pain or serious discomfort for the last month and a half. Each time one pain subsides, another pops up. The biopsy pain faded just in time for surgery. Then as the incision stopped hurting, I discovered it was masking the lymph-node pain in my arm. As that faded, my port went in, and now I feel a sharp burning sensation anytime it's touched, even lightly. I wonder if chemo hurts.

My oncologist wrote a prescription for a wig. I got a kick out of it; I was going to make copies and frame it for Wade's upcoming pottery show.

But as it turns out, my insurance won't pay for a wig, even with a prescription. So instead of making copies, I'll frame the original for Wade's show. Still, it's hard to complain about insurance not covering a wig when they're covering the giant expense of chemotherapy.

Marshmallow-Free Camp Chemo
Friday, October 19, 2007, 8:18 p.m.

When Wade and I arrived for Camp Chemo, we were led to a small conference room where one older, retired couple had already arrived. The wife was in for colon cancer. After the nurse started a video, the woman with lung cancer I'd met in the waiting room a few weeks ago came in, wheeling her oxygen tank behind her. So three patients, two spouses. The class consisted of a twenty-five-minute video followed by a question-and-answer session with the nurse. She had our charts so she could answer questions specific to our individual cases.

From the video, we learned: we'll be tired. Really, really tired. A healthy diet of small, frequent meals helps control nausea. Sex during chemo requires a condom because the medicine can transfer through body fluids. Eeeeewww!

From the nurse, we learned: my hair will be gone about two or three weeks after the first treatment. A private room is usually available for chemo if the appointment is early in the day. Stay on top of the nausea medication—take it as soon as symptoms start, or it's impossible to keep even a pill down.

Alas, Camp Chemo had no campfire, no singing, and no roasting of marshmallows.

The only fun part was visiting the American Cancer Society wig room. There I picked up a free wig. I'll miss having my real hair, because I love it. It's dark brown and very long, nearly to my elbows. But it will be interesting to look a bit different for a while. Turns out I look terrible as a blonde and even worse as a redhead. Guess I was born to be brunette. Now I'll never know if blondes have more fun. Darn.

Each time a doctor or nurse talks about my chemo, they give me a look like, "This TAC is going to be bad. These are big guns." This probably should make me nervous, but I feel like it's just a bigger challenge, as if they're betting me to fall apart during the treatment. And I refuse.

Lately, it occurs to me that technically there's no medical evidence that any cancer remains in my body. I could be cured, but there's no way to know. So I'm choosing to think of the chemo, radiation, and (afterward) tamoxifen as preventative medicine to double-check that the cancer is all gone. I'm choosing to think of myself as a survivor. I believe in the power of the words. I'm going to start saying "I had breast cancer" in the past tense, instead of "I have breast cancer" in the present tense.

I don't know much about the causes of cancer, but I know the major ones aren't in play here: I have no family history; I don't drink; I don't smoke; I get plenty of exercise; I don't drink caffeine or eat red meat. Still, this afternoon, I went to the organic grocery store to delete a few possible cancer agents from my life. I bought some deodorant made from natural mineral salts. I'll let you know how that works tomorrow after I go to the gym. I also got a metal water bottle from Switzerland, which should be healthier than drinking from plastic. Processed soy—not tofu, but soy in powder form like in energy bars—has already been eliminated from my diet. That's because my cancer is estrogen receptive, meaning the cancer is fueled by estrogen, and processed soy is thought to have high estrogenicity. Say that five times fast.

Camp Chemo Packing List
Sunday, October 21, 2007, 10:50 p.m.

What do you get when you take two lawyers, an auditor, and a corporate consultant? A really clean house. And a fantastic meal. No joke. Four friends spent two hours cleaning my house. That's eight hours of cleaning, and our house hasn't been this sparkling in years! The nesting for chemotherapy is complete.

So many other gifts arrived this weekend. Some tangible: a book for Vivian to read, write, and draw about experiencing illness in her family; and also for Vivian, a groovy pink nightlight; for our family, we received a delicious organic veggie and chicken stew; gift certificates to our favorite grocery stores and cards wishing us well. Other gifts were intangible but just as real: prayers; phone calls from friends; kind words written on my CaringBridge page. We also had some fun this weekend, Wade and I ate a spicy Thai meal at a restaurant. He took Vivian to the Children's Theater, while I watched Jackson play with Play-Doh for the very first time—no doubt the start of a beautiful (and possibly delicious) relationship.

Tomorrow is my first chemotherapy session. Lots of confusion over what to wear. If this was an actual Camp Chemo, there would be a packing list. It's past 10:00 p.m., and on typical days, I would've set out the next day's clothes by now. For chemo, should I don my regular "procedure wear" of black, loose-fitting drawstring gym pants, a V-neck T-shirt (for ease of port access near my collarbone), my gray zip-up sweater, with red tennies? Or should I come up with something more festive? Perhaps a scarf in my hair? Which reminds me . . .

I got my hair cut yesterday! I love it! My stylist is brilliant. It's a very short messy bob with loads of bangs. This whole experience will make me way more adventurous with hairstyles in the future. Vivian was there for the cut, and she squealed with shock and delight as my two long ponytails were cut for Locks of Love.

Today, I took four tablets of Dexamethasone, a corticosteroid, to prepare for tomorrow's trip to the fun house. Then, once I get home, I'll take two other meds for nausea. After reading the instructions from the pharmacy, I just have to share the hilarious (only if they don't actually happen to anyone) side effects. Here's my disclaimer to the disclaimers, if you are easily grossed out or offended, cover your ears for the next paragraph.

In addition to the typical side effects, including headache, muscle aches, fever, dizziness, sore throat, and painful erection, these medications have some really creative ones that I've not seen before—inability to move eyes, twitching or twisting movements, masklike face (what, like too-much-makeup mask? Halloween mask? Mardi Gras mask?), shuffling walk, stiff arms, puffing of cheeks, lip smacking or puckering, personality changes, and—my favorite—vomit that looks like coffee grounds. Who writes this stuff?!

My dream job used to be thinking up names for nail polishes and eye shadows: Eternal Pink, Probably Willow, Tomorrow Blue. Now my dream job is thinking up side effects for medications: fear of small objects, rattling bones, inability to walk backward, thirst for vengeance.

Pray for me tomorrow morning; I go in at 8:30, and chemo should take about four hours. Luckily, Wade is coming with me, and they have cookies in the lobby, so at least I have something to look forward to.

First Chemo

Monday, October 22, 2007, 8:15 p.m.

Last night, I got only three hours of sleep. Not only the anxiety of today's chemo kept me up, but Jackson is suffering from a terrible cold, so he was really restless. The upside of my insomnia is that I finished reading *When Bad Things Happen to Good People* by Rabbi Harold S. Kushner. Needless to say, it gave me an interesting theological perspective on illness and some new ways to think about my situation. I highly recommend this book to everyone.

The chemotherapy itself was painless and actually pretty boring. At first, I thought it was silly for Wade to take the morning off work to just sit around with me for four hours. But I was so happy to have him there. The instructions the nurse gave about the medications were confusing and overwhelming, but Wade took good notes. Just having him in the room was comforting.

Then late this afternoon, I started to feel nauseous and exhausted. Maybe the result of a lack of sleep more than chemo. I wanted to work, or do something, but I felt rotten. Jackson's cold is terrible, so despite having my mom, Ernestine (Ernie for short), there to help, he was fussy all afternoon. Vivian was upset about her after-school plans going awry. Poor Wade is drained from trying to hold us all together.

When I tried to get Jackson to sleep, he didn't want his bottle or his Binky. Instead, he asked to nurse for the first time since the biopsy. Normally, when a baby is ill, the best thing is to nurse for the added immunity. It broke my heart to say no and to listen to him cry.

After Jackson finally fell asleep and Vivian was in the bath, Wade and I cried together over this whole thing for the very first time since the diagnosis. The trigger was me saying, "I just want our normal lives back." It's making me tear up again right now. Vivian kept calling for me from the bathtub, and I still had tears in my eyes when I came in, so I told her I was feeling overwhelmed and sad. She said she was feeling the same way. Then she started singing a song we used to sing when she was a toddler.

Skida-ma-rink-ee-dink-ee-dink, skida-ma-rink-ee-doo, I love you,
Skida-ma-rink-ee-dink-ee-dink, skida-ma-rink-ee-doo, I love you.
I love you in the morning and in the afternoon,
I love you in the evening and underneath the moon,
Oh, skida-ma-rink-ee-dink-ee-dink,
Skida-ma-rink-ee-doo, I love you!

That made me cry even more—and then giggle as she splashed me.

In my rational mind, I count the blessings of our family life and the support from family and friends in the past month and a half. In my emotional mind, I want my body back, I want my long brunette hair back, I want my dream of living to one hundred years old back. Mostly, I want to chicken out on this whole chemotherapy deal and quit. But I guess you can't call in sick to chemo.

One of the nausea medications, Ativan—a.k.a. lorazepam—will also help me sleep. That pill is calling my name right now. A good twelve hours of shut-eye should make me a new woman. Despite today's tears, I'm looking forward to tomorrow, a new day.

Asleep for Days
Thursday, October 25, 2007, 9:07 p.m.

Wade, the husband, writing. Here we are at the end of a beautiful October evening. Jackson and Vivian are both sleeping comfortably and peacefully. Camille is also sleeping. In fact, she has been since about 5:00 p.m. on Tuesday. Of course she wakes periodically to drink water or apple juice, and when she does, amazingly, her eyes are always bright and cheery, and she is quick to smile. She's had no appetite to speak of since Monday afternoon. Perhaps a saltine or two, but that's been about it.

So imagine my surprise when she calls me tonight during Vivian's piano lesson to ask me to pick up some McDonald's french fries with ketchup. She came out to the table to join us and ate a little bit of the bun from my Filet-O-Fish. That's weird, right? Wake up after two and a half days longing for McD's?

The good thing I realized today is that the mystery of Camp Chemo is gone. We now know what to expect during the next four months, and that's comforting. I no longer worry about her body being ravaged with gut-cramping vomiting spells. I'm not concerned about shielding the kids from her, for their emotional protection. (However, I do shield her from them, of course, because as we all know they are festering, moldering, germ-laden petri dishes looking for their next host [i.e., parent] to infect.) I can handle her sleeping for days; that's fairly simple compared to what I was anticipating.

I guess preparing for the worst is a blessing, because now I feel good—no, not good, but OK about what's to come. Don't get me wrong; we'll definitely still need your support whether it be prayers, energy, karma, or dare I say food—it's just really nice to see her asleep and at peace in that sleep, rather than the various unpleasant alternatives.

Thanks for listening. You sleep well too.

Wade

Pancakes

Saturday, October 27, 2007, 9:56 a.m.

The delicious pancakes Wade made this morning marked my first breakfast since Monday. My, how time flies when you don't eat or drink. Dehydration landed me in the clinic for eight hours yesterday to get replenished with IV fluids. I'm still really tired, but at least now, I can get up to do more than just go to the bathroom. Still not in the mood to socialize much. I know that's been hard on people calling to send good wishes.

It's frustrating to be feeling better but still not even close to 50 percent power yet. At least we know now the difference between chemo and dehydration, the latter of which can be prevented pretty easily. I made some paper bottles so Vivian can help me keep track of how much fluid I'm getting, and it's a little math lesson to boot. She's been a super trooper.

We finally watched *E. T.* last night. We've been trying to get Vivian to see it for over a year, but she was afraid it would be too scary. We wanted her to see it because she looks so much like Drew Barrymore at that age. Vivian loved the character E.T., and even after I left the movie for bed, I could hear her squealing and screaming with delight.

All of your love and well wishes are making a world of difference in these dark days. They're like cheerful care packages arriving at Camp Chemo.

Annoyed

Sunday, October 28, 2007, 8:09 p.m.

Energy conservation is the phrase of the day. I have the ambition to do so many things, but my body just doesn't have the energy for it all.

The most beautiful thing about the past few days is that my dreamless sleep was at last replaced by dreams once again. And they've been wonderful, colorful, glorious dreams where I've been able to run around with the kids, go to fun classes, do theater games, hear music, make art, see shows, and more. Each nap has been rewarded by more of these great dreams. In one series of dreams, we vacationed in the same spot for three years in a row and had a blast seeing our vacation friends every year. As night starts to fall, I'm looking forward to going back into dreamland tonight.

Today, I took a long, long walk up to the corner store with Wade (four blocks round trip) in the cool, crisp air. It was the most exercise I've had since Monday, and it felt great. No medications today made for a pretty clear head, and it was nice to have some conversations. I was also able to eat a large breakfast of three pancakes with applesauce, a lunch of rice and pizza, and, well, at dinner, I was back to "what's the minimum amount I can ingest without angering the stomach gods?" I'm not sure why after eating breakfast and lunch it's difficult to eat dinner. Maybe my stomach is still getting used to food again.

As I was writing, Vivian said, "This breast cancer is a lot worse than I'd thought it would be." When we questioned her, she said, "Mom's been back and forth and back and forth to bed and the hospital." When we asked how she feels about it all, she said, "Annoyed." Ditto on that, little darling.

I hesitate to write too much about the kids in these posts from Camp Chemo because this is part of their story too, and someday they'll tell their own story about this time in our lives—if it's something they even remember. Hopefully, it will be nothing more than an annoying speed bump. A small distraction that got in the way of our family's plans for a short time.

Dog Nose
Tuesday, October 30, 2007, 6:54 a.m.

During the first trimester of pregnancy, it's been reported that the olfactory sense of a pregnant woman is stronger than that of a dog. That was true for me when I was carrying both kids. Chemotherapy is similar. The total exhaustion of the initial chemo is passing, and the nausea is slowing down, but my canine sense of smell is going strong. Yesterday I went into the office for just a few minutes, and the immediate assault of food smells drifting from the office kitchen nearly drove me over the edge. It was really hard to be there. Plus, it's difficult to act normal (energetic, excited, interested) when you're not feeling well. I was able to make some phone calls and have a few e-mail exchanges yesterday from home. It's amazing how easy it is to fake feeling well on the phone.

Another experience now has me shopping for airsickness bags online. Thank God Wade was driving me home from work (since I still don't yet feel safe driving), because I kept being assaulted by every smell. The stench of a diesel truck sent me over the edge, and I lost my lunch just a few blocks from home. I couldn't get the car door open quite in time. Let's just say that I really wish we'd been driving a rental car.

I'll be working from home again today. The smell of Wade's coffee is making me crazy this morning. When I was pregnant, I banned the use of the coffeemaker in our home, and Wade had to buy coffee on his way to work. It may come to that again. Thank goodness I never picked up the coffee habit. If I had, I'd be in big trouble now.

Yesterday, my white counts were checked, and while they are down, as expected, they're not low enough to require additional medicine. Phew. Working from home is a great option, though it makes me nervous because Jackson has been fighting a bad cold for over a week. My mom will do her best to keep him away from me today, which she's been doing successfully for a week already. Having Mom around to help is priceless.

Last night at bedtime, Vivian asked if children can get breast cancer. I said no and explained the role of estrogen. I explained when she's a young adult, she'll get extra preventative tests because of my cancer. She asked if men can get breast cancer, and I explained yes. We talked about the causes of cancer and how my doctor isn't sure why I got it. We talked about generally accepted healthy lifestyles. Vivian wonders if drinking a little bit of coffee occasionally may have caused my cancer. Her insightful questions tell me that she has the brains and persistence to help cure this lousy disease someday.

Still having the most beautiful dreams at night. Can't remember the details right now, but they're all colorful and filled with friends, family, and parties—in a word, heaven. Sweet dreams to you.

Halloweenie Roast
Wednesday, October 31, 2007, 9:29 p.m.

I feel the best kind of exhausted right now. It's a true exhaustion from a long, pleasant day, not from being sick. Halloween couldn't have been more perfect. Vivian dressed as a beautiful gypsy. Jackson dressed as a hobo, but after putting on the patched shirt, black greasepaint eyebrows, beard, and mustache, I thought he looked more like Chuck Norris dressed as a rodeo clown for a bad episode of *Walker, Texas Ranger.*

For the last four years, we've hosted a Halloweenie Roast for the neighborhood kids. We never doubted we'd go ahead with the party this year. It's the one party you can have and not clean the house, because the whole party is outside. We simply put a table in the front yard, cook hot dogs in a Crock-Pot, set out hot dog buns, ketchup, mustard, chips, and juice boxes, and call it a party. There's nothing Martha Stewart about it. In fact, Martha Stewart would probably find it disgraceful.

Men, skip this paragraph if you're squeamish. But alas, after running around with the kids from door to door and feeling really great tonight (Vivian even commented, "Mom, you seem totally fine tonight"), I got back to the house, and *bam*—like some memento mori, I realized my period was starting again for the second time in two weeks. How valiant that nature makes these last-ditch attempts to propagate the species. While my body is being poisoned, my reproductive system hurries for one last offspring. I've cycled a perfect twenty-eight days since age ten—and yes, starting at ten was traumatic. Truth be told, that's a leading probable cause for my breast cancer. My periods started early in life, and I waited until late in life to have children. Those are the only two risk factors I've been able to identify that apply to me.

Tomorrow is a religious holiday, one of my favorites—All Saints' Day. I love that it's traditionally celebrated in Mexico as the Day of the Dead. Like Halloween, the Day of the Dead involves candy (shaped into skulls), but also visits to grave sites to remember relatives who have died, and you bring them candy too. It makes death seem less scary, a more natural part of life. Not that I'm planning on passing over anytime soon—quite the contrary; I have plenty of living to do.

As you rise to All Saints' Day tomorrow, may you remember those who have gone before you, those without whom you wouldn't be here or without whom you wouldn't be you. May you notice the saints living among you, and may you be a saint to someone in need as so many have been to me in this time of need.

On the Glass

Saturday, November 3, 2007, 11:58 p.m.

You know that expression "I'll sleep when I'm dead"? Lately, I'm so hyper—up past my bedtime and loving life. It's like my own "I'll rest during chemo week" philosophy.

Tonight was a blast. We got a babysitter because a friend gave us free hockey tickets. The Minnesota Wild won, my favorite player, Derek Boogaard, got into two fights, and here's the best part—we spent the last two periods *on the glass*! Now if you're not into hockey, let me explain. It's like box seats at the opera, only better because it's the front row, and you can bang on the Plexiglas at the players. You can't do that at the opera.

Cancer has somehow made me more daring. And why not? I've looked the grim reaper in the face and given him the middle finger. Tonight, Wade was my brilliant accomplice: after the first period in our nosebleed seats, we snuck down onto the main level into two empty seats on the glass that we'd noticed from above. I'm not sure if it's illegal or just immoral, but wow, was it worth the risk. That's upgrading from (free) $35 tickets to $225 seats. This new relationship with risk is an attribute I can embrace.

My relationship with money has also been changing lately. Sometimes I'm way more frugal than I was before because, oh my, we really should be more responsible with our money. Other times, I'm more likely to treat myself—for example, tonight I spent the three dollars for the glossy hockey program, which I love. We also stopped at a cute diner afterward for apple pie and hash browns—ten delicious dollars we didn't need to spend, but you're buying the experience more than the food.

Chemo Dread

Tuesday, November 6, 2007, 3:44 p.m.

Have you ever suffered from what I call Sunday sickness? It happens on Sunday evening when you realize, "Crap, I have to go to work tomorrow morning, and I really don't want to." It's anxiety accompanied by a tummy ache and an overwhelming sense of dread. Premature Sunday sickness is a good analogy for what I started to feel this afternoon—an overwhelming sense of dread for next Monday, when I go in for my second chemo. I called a breast cancer survivor who is about six weeks ahead of me in her chemo. She told me she once got physically ill just thinking about her next clinic visit. Good to know this anxiety is normal.

Handfuls of Hair

Thursday, November 8, 2007, 9:14 p.m.

Yesterday, a few fashionistas at work looked at my wig and gave me some feedback. I now feel like I can wear my short, brown wig to work and anywhere else with confidence when the time comes. The office scarf expert loaned me a collection of beautiful scarves and taught me how to do that movie star head wrap that's so glam. Then, today, a friend bought me another wig, a cute, dark-brown bob. While I'm not that into fashion and don't like to spend money on clothes, I'm sure glad to have hip friends so I can get good advice.

Dr. Anderson, my oncologist, told me my hair would start to fall out within two or three weeks of my first treatment. Monday was exactly two weeks, and in the shower, while shampooing, I got a handful of hair. Each day, more falls out. My hair is very thick, so once I have it dried and styled, the loss isn't noticeable yet, but I'm glad to be prepared with my wigs because their time is coming soon.

Physically, my scalp is starting to hurt. It feels like something is pulling on it. If you've ever worn a tight ponytail and then let it out at the end of the day, it's that feeling. But the feeling is all over my entire scalp. I'm curious about the scientific explanation for this strange sensation.

Lately, I'm feeling good physically but been having a hard time emotionally. During the day, I'm OK, but around 7:00 or 8:00 p.m. I fall into a bad mood and get crabby with the kids. I've also been feeling anxious and depressed all at once, which is a strange combination of emotions for me.

I'm freaked out at work, because I'm taking time off after chemo and for Thanksgiving, so I'm only working one day a week for the next two weeks. It isn't enough time to get much done! My boss, Barb, and my very generous coworkers are willing to help, so I'll be spending most of my time tomorrow and Monday on specific instructions of what they can do to help when I'm out of the office. It's really hard to let go, because I like my job, and I have so much control at the office that I don't have with my healing.

Skinhead

Saturday, November 10, 2007, 9:07 p.m.

Today, I asked Wade to shave my head. My hair was falling out when I touched it. My shedding was going to make such a mess that keeping the remaining hair just wasn't worth it. Luckily, Wade's grooming preference means he's an experienced head shaver. He knew exactly what to do. Vivian was there, but about halfway through the shaving, she left the room. When she saw me without my hair, she just said it looked weird. She wanted me to put on my wig immediately.

Wade, on the other hand, thought it was cool to see me as a skinhead. He thinks I should just buy some punk band T-shirts and take on a new persona.

I was surprised to see how much of my hair is pure white. About a year ago, I started using hair dye to cover it. Now, I'm about 25 percent white. I don't look as bad without hair as I thought I might, just different. My eyes look much larger, and I definitely appear shorter. If it were more socially acceptable for women to go bald, I'd probably go without a wig more often. But it's getting close to winter, so soon it'll be too cold for that, anyway.

The most upsetting part of the whole process was seeing all my hair in the trash can. There was something startling and sad about that. But having no hair is weirdly liberating. Once my hair starts to grow back, I might experiment with short styles for a while until I get bored and want long hair again.

I wore the wig over to our friends' house for dinner but was happy to remove it at home—wigs really itch. I noticed that when I'd smile or laugh, the wig felt weird on my head.

Later this evening, I experimented with false eyelashes. In a way, I'm more upset about losing my eyebrows and eyelashes; they're more difficult to replace than hair. The eyelashes will take considerable practice before they look even remotely unlike a drag queen's prop.

Wig Decisions
Sunday, November 11, 2007, 10:24 p.m.

My baldness continues to be an issue for Vivian. She's such a girlie girl, and she loves long hair, so this is really tough for her. Out of respect for her, I wore a wig to church today. Wow, did it itch! I want to order a cap for my head to wear under the wig to prevent itchiness. Later this afternoon, Vivian said it's OK to wear a head scarf out of the house, which is much more comfortable. When I'm at the house alone or at the office without client appointments, I might go without a head covering, because it's so much more comfortable. Maybe once my hair has completely fallen out, my scalp won't be so sensitive, but right now, it's very uncomfortable. I want to balance my discomfort with how people feel about seeing me without hair. While I'm cool with no hair, others may find it upsetting. We'll see.

My mom is unsettled by seeing me without hair. Growing up as an only child with a single parent, our relationship often felt more like siblings. We rarely argued, but one subject of ongoing disagreement was my hair. I wanted it long; my mom preferred it short. Truth be told, short hair does suit my face better, but I love the look of long hair. About half of my young life, it was long; about half the time, it was short. That represents our great ability to compromise.

Wade is still going on and on about how great I look without hair, which is cool to hear from the man I love. He rocks.

I'm highly motivated to drink a ton of water and POWERADE and eat a ton of popsicles and chipped ice in the next week to get my two liters in each day. The source of my motivation? Another pair of free Minnesota Wild hockey tickets for Sunday night. Last chemo round, I was too weak on Sunday to go anywhere but up the block. I think the dehydration, not the chemo, was the problem. We booked a babysitter for the hockey game either way. If I'm not well enough to attend the game, I won't be well enough to stay home alone with two kids. With each sip of POWERADE, I'll be thinking about sneaking into a seat on the glass. Look for me on the Jumbotron!

Game Over

Monday, November 12, 2007, 6:51 p.m.

During chemo today, I was surrounded by my "cozy angels"—a double-fleece blanket from a church friend, a shawl my neighbor knitted for me, and a cap my mother-in-law, Beckie, knitted for me. The chemo room is cold, so it was nice to be warm this time. I felt in good spirits and even chatted with several other patients. The nurses were, as always, wonderful.

Dr. Anderson was amazed at my white blood counts. He showed me how high they've remained and said that normally during chemo they go way down. I told him I'm an overachiever, so I love to hear that news!

The last time I saw him, he explained that with chemo and radiation, we're going after a cure. But if the cancer metastasizes from my breast to anywhere else in my body—like bones, liver, or lung—they can only "prolong life." This had been troubling me, so today I asked what it would mean to me if the cancer were to metastasize. He summed it up in two words: game over. If the cancer metastasizes, I will die of cancer. It means

I'll have to do chemo for the rest of my life. Gulp. Now I understand why people are so afraid of cancer returning, metastasizing. I got teary and said that I've always wanted to be an old lady someday. He told me that I can be. He said I could live to be seventy, eighty, even ninety. This surprised me because I've only heard of ten-, fifteen-, and twenty-year breast cancer survivors. Maybe the treatment is much better now.

While part of me wants to continue healthy behaviors, another part feels like it didn't work in the past, so what's the point? That's a good example of the sort of internal conflicts I'm struggling with these days. Dr. Anderson said not to worry about anything past my next treatment in three weeks. His advice: "Don't lose your cool." That's my new mantra.

Vivian's feelings teacher (that's what she calls the school social worker) gave her a feelings book where she can write down her emotions. I read it, and yikes, she's very sad about my chemo and worried about me. She's having a hard time with my shaved head. Now that my hair is gone, it's impossible to forget that this thing is happening. For all of us.

These days, I'm off to bed when the kids go to bed. I've decided to embrace rest, rather than fight it like I did last time around. Good night.

Sleeping Off the Chemo
Friday, November 16, 2007, 9:15 p.m.

Wade here. As you can probably guess, Camille has had a bit of a hard week, although better than last time. She's been sleeping a lot but eating more and staying on top of her fluids a little better this time. The help her mother has given us this week has been priceless. I've been able to work almost a full schedule, and Jackson seems really happy hanging out with grandma. Vivian is doing much better this time, as well.

Thanks to those of you who supplied all the food this week and last week. Having the dinner rush taken care of has definitely relieved a significant amount of pressure. I've also posted pictures of Camille with her beautiful shaved head. She's AWESOME.

Wade

Rock Bottom

Saturday, November 17, 2007, 8:32 a.m.

Finally, I'm starting to descend from the chemo fog I've been in for the past week. Yesterday, I hit rock bottom. I felt I couldn't go on any longer. Wade and I sat outside for a while as Jackson slept indoors with the baby monitor safely listening to him. While I hate to admit it, I was feeling suicidal. I wouldn't ever actually do it. It's just something that seems like the best alternative to how I'm feeling. I keep thinking that if I died, it would be just fine. It would be peaceful. When I feel so ill I can't remember what it's like to feel well, and I lose all hope that I'll ever feel better . . . death becomes the ultimate escape. After talking with Wade, we went indoors, and I called my nurse and doctor. They confirmed physical reasons I was feeling so emotionally low.

After I described to the nurse how terrible I felt, she gave me the green light to take Ativan, which allows me to sleep soundly. Thank goodness. But then after I got off the phone, Wade and I realized the baby monitor receiver was still outside—broadcasting every private and scary word to the entire neighborhood. You laugh or you cry, right?

Resting

Tuesday, November 20, 2007, 7:03 a.m.

Rest has been my focus for the last few days. Saturday and Sunday nights, I couldn't settle down until after 1:00 a.m. I've always needed a full eight hours of sleep, so late nights aren't sustainable for more than a day or two. Plus, I need more rest these days to relax my sore muscles and joints. Last night, I took an Epsom salts bath, which helped relieve the pain, and then I went directly to bed. Today, I'm rested, and my body feels much better.

Yesterday, I finally told Shelly, my oldest and dearest friend, about my diagnosis. After the original surgery, we played a few rounds of phone tag, but then I somehow lost her cell number, which still boggles my mind.

On some level, I think I was dreading the conversation because I knew she'd be deeply upset. Her father died recently from cancer.

Speaking with her, I realized it's time to look squarely at my feelings, acknowledge them, deal with them, and move on. I was trying to be cheerful by comforting her about my condition when she said that it's OK to be angry, to feel faithless—and working through those feelings is important, because it's inevitable that they'll come up. Shelly helped me realize that I don't need to protect others or myself from difficult feelings. Good advice.

Giving Thanks

Thanksgiving Day, Thursday, November 22, 2007, 7:19 p.m.

Happy Thanksgiving! What am I thankful for this year?

My health. Believe it or not, despite my recent brush with cancer, I'm so happy to possess overall good health.

My eyebrows and eyelashes. They're thinning, but still there. Losing my hair can be covered with wigs or scarves, but living without brows and lashes will make me look even more like a cancer patient, which I dread.

Two-minute showers. And half of that time is standing around enjoying the water! With no shampooing, conditioning, or shaving, showers are a snap these days.

Happy, healthy children. Need I say more?

A mate who adores me. He really does, and he shows me daily. And I love him more each day!

All the best to your family this Thanksgiving.

Anne

Friday, November 23, 2007, 2:26 p.m.

Black Friday. Shopping craziness. I wore Anne to the mall today. Who is Anne? She's an upstanding citizen, pays her bills on time, eats her veggies, and always remembers to write a thank-you note. Anne is my short, brunette wig. She's the day-to-day workhorse I've been wearing to the office. With her, I can go anywhere without drawing attention to my head. Just like lipstick and nail polish colors, wigs come with a name, usually a woman's name.

Yesterday, I introduced Anne to our extended family in Iowa. This is our first visit since I've lost my hair. Today, I wore her to the mall with my niece, Amanda (she was up at 3:30 a.m. to start her Black Friday shopping. People in Iowa are early risers!) Vivian and I joined Amanda at 6:30. I promised Vivian one treat, which she bought at Claire's, the kid's accessory store at the mall. Later in the day, I returned to Claire's to buy a Christmas present for Vivian, this time wearing just a bandana on my head. The clerk who helped us early in the morning was still there, and I thought it was a perfect opportunity for an objective response. I said, "Hi, I was in early this morning, but I was wearing a wig. Now I have this bandana," so she'd recognize me. She said, "I never would've guessed that was a wig. It really looked real. Wow, I can't believe it." That was good confirmation that at least to a complete stranger, Anne is doing her job—making sure I don't look strange.

Speaking of looking strange, our house doesn't have a full-length mirror in the bathroom or bedroom, but when we visit Iowa, where there's a wall of full-length mirrors in the bathroom, I can't help but . . . notice things. With my bald head, I resemble a mannequin. The scar over my right breast isn't a straight line; it's curved slightly, like an upside-down U. It reminds me of an eyebrow. When I lift my right arm, it goes into a coy arch, like it belongs to Scarlett O'Hara. Together, all six scars (four from the biopsy and surgery on the right side, two from the port on the left) form a shape much like the Little Dipper. Just one more little scar near the center of my breastbone would complete the constellation.

Chemo Dread Again
Wednesday, November 28, 2007, 7:36 a.m.

This morning, I woke to Jackson throwing socks at me and crawling on my head. I didn't want to get up but didn't have much choice. Now he's rolling up his little sleeves and getting to work riding his "bike"—a four-wheeled scooter.

In the last few days, I've been feeling my mental health deteriorating. It's more and more difficult to feel optimistic because I've been worrying about so many things. Yesterday morning, I had a good cry in one of my bosses' office. Despite tons of support at work, I know it could take a year to get my billing (and income) back up to where I want after all my treatments are done. Still, I work at a nonprofit and am happy that even if my income suffers, my work is supporting a greater good.

I'm worried about my next chemo. It's not until next week, but already I'm dreading it. Even going to the clinic these past two Mondays for my blood draws has required a lot of courage to pull myself through the clinic doors. It's stressful to see how other people later in treatment are doing. One of my chemo buddies (dubbed my "chemo sabe," à la *The Lone Ranger,* by our mutual friend Joe) has been barred from chemo treatments two weeks in a row due to low white counts. There's nothing worse than psyching yourself up to be out of work for a week, only to be told you have to wait another week for chemo.

On Friday, I'll see a psychologist with experience working with oncology patients. My hope is to gain some ideas on how to deal with this ever-changing journey.

Last night, we put up the (artificial) Christmas tree. It's from a friend who used to work with me at an alternative music radio station in the 1990s. Courtney Love knocked over that very tree on stage during their holiday music show. Even though I want to get rid of it and go back to having a real tree, its unusual provenance makes it hard to let it go.

Now Jackson is on my lap and in need of kisses. Gotta go.

Psychological Help

Friday, November 30, 2007, 10:40 p.m.

Today, I received good ideas and comfort from the psychologist. She reminded me that in the present moment, I am safe. That's something I'll be able to use when I start to worry. She also reminded me that chemo drugs are powerful and they are indeed drugs, so it's no wonder my mental health isn't quite what it used to be. After meeting with her, I have hope that next week's chemo recovery will go even better than the last two sessions.

Lately, I've been thinking of myself as a moth drawn to a light—I feel an urgent need to create, live, love. The light both terrifies and comforts me. I worry that drawing closer to it can only mean my journey in this existence is ending.

Pottery Sale

Sunday, December 2, 2007, 9:32 p.m.

The day before Thanksgiving, I started a news fast, and it's been really nice. As a result, though, it was Friday afternoon before I started to hear from family and friends that the first snowstorm of the year was going to dump six to eight inches of snow on the day of Wade's pottery and painting sale.

Sure enough, on Saturday morning, it looked like a snow globe outside our window. The twelve-minute drive over to the sale location took a good twenty-five minutes, and we saw one car in the ditch alongside the freeway.

It seemed Mother Nature was conspiring against us. Then Wade reminded me of something from when we used to do outdoor art fairs. Bad weather often brings out the best buyers. Our theory is that if someone braves bad weather, that person doesn't want to go home empty-handed. They want something to show for their trouble.

This definitely proved true for our art sale yesterday. We made much more money than we normally make in a three-day art fair! We were amazed at how many people came. Some of my mom's friends came from far-flung suburbs, forty-five minutes away in good weather. My cousin Kelsey from New Mexico won the prize for longest trek. What a great surprise to see her! It was so delightful to talk with people I haven't seen in years. One thirty-year breast cancer survivor gave me wonderful sense of hope by sharing that her cancer has never returned.

In addition to selling a lot of Wade's pottery, I sold a few dozen Camp Chemo T-shirts! Wade also sold two paintings. They went at the eleventh hour. It's always a little difficult to see paintings go, but I feel good knowing they'll be loved and enjoyed by people outside our house too.

Vivian had a blast. More than a dozen of her friends showed up, so it was a nonstop party for her. She was so well behaved; she was a joy to be around. My mom watched over Jackson, who was darling until he got crabby around naptime.

My spirits are high going into my third round of chemo tomorrow morning. While I don't want to feel sick, my psychologist provided several good thoughts and visualizations to bring into the next few days.

At one point during my time in bed after my last round, I was crying out to God for help, just like David did in so many of the psalms. So I decided that Psalm 46 would be my inspiration during this round:

> *God is our refuge and strength, a very present help in trouble.*
> *Therefore we will not fear, though the earth be moved, and though the mountains be toppled into the depths of the sea;*
> *Though its waters rage and foam, and though the mountains tremble at its tumult.*
> *The Lord of hosts is with us; the God of Jacob is our stronghold.*

I'll keep the psalm close to my heart and in the drawer of my bedside stand to remember that strength is just a prayer (or a loud cry) away.

I'll also keep two images of Vivian in my mind from today—in her choir robe during her church children's choir performance, and in her pretty red-and-white costume during her Swedish folk dance. (Did I mention this is Minnesota?)

Chemo Introvert
Wednesday, December 5, 2007, 9:26 a.m.

So far, this round of treatment is going much better than the first two. It surprises me because the side effects should be cumulative, which I expect would make them worse with each treatment. This time, I'm only taking the expensive antinausea drugs, rather than mixing in the cheaper ones, so that's helping. Today, I'll run out of the more expensive pills, though, so I wonder if I'll feel worse tomorrow. The cheaper drugs make my mind foggy.

I have no interest in the world outside my house during the week after a chemo treatment. Talking on the phone, listening to the radio, watching TV, reading the paper—none of those activities appeal to me. And I've felt this way after each one. It's so strange for me, a lifelong extrovert, to shy away from human interaction.

Another Week Asleep
Sunday, December 9, 2007, 7:22 p.m.

In addition to sleeping nine to ten hours at night, I've been taking two naps each day lasting three or four hours each. Pretty much a cat's sleep schedule.

I'm not sure if it was all the sleep Monday through Friday or if it's something else, but I haven't been sleeping well the past two nights. I tried taking a nap today, but it was like naps when I was a preschooler. My exhausted single-parent mom would say, "Take a nap!" and I'd just lie in bed, wide awake, waiting for naptime to be over.

During the week I slept, life went on. Vivian attended the church Christmas party with another family. Jackson fell off a chair and got his first stitches in the ER. Vivian attended a dance performance with neighbors. Jackson got his first haircut. Right now, Wade is playing Matchbox cars with Jackson and the neighbor kids.

On Friday, I kept feeling that our house is so stale. Being cooped up for days at a time in winter is a surefire way to get really sick of your decor. I've spent much of my drive time this weekend keeping an eye out for houses for sale. It would be so nice when this is all over to just start all over again.

I'm exhausted from this whole journey. I thought that being halfway through chemo would be a joyful moment. It isn't. This illness is getting boring and old. I want my old life again. I want to pretend that none of this ever happened.

Today, Wade suggested I go to the gym, so I did. I've only been a few times since surgery, and this is the first time since my hair fell out. I wore a blue bandana on my head. There's this unwritten code at the gym that you don't talk to anyone unless you know them from outside the gym. So there was no opportunity to explain to all the familiar faces what happened to me, why I have no hair under that bandana.

Normally, when I go to the gym, I feel good about doing something active to improve my health and future. But I felt like a failure today, because despite my efforts at healthy living, I still wasn't able to prevent this illness.

The feeling of failure followed me from the gym to the grocery store. I felt like I was being judged—maybe that white bread or mac and cheese in my cart was the reason for the cancer. A twenty-two-year breast cancer survivor approached me in the cookie aisle to give me some encouragement. It was nice to talk with her, but on the other hand, it was a bummer to be acknowledged only for my lack of hair.

I know many of the thoughts I'm having are irrational.

Tonight, our next-door neighbor brought dinner and joined us for the meal. Sometimes having an extended conversation *not* about how I'm feeling is just what the doctor ordered.

Two States of Being

Tuesday, December 11, 2007, 8:53 p.m.

Today was my first day back to work after this round. It's so good to be back to the land of the living!

Part of the difficulty I'm having seems related to the two very distinct states I experience these days. The chemo state is very unlike my normal life. During the four or five days after chemo, I'm so annoyed that most of my hours are spent sleeping. And when I'm awake, I'm not myself. I want no contact with the world. I'm realizing that's just how the drugs affect me, and I can't hope to change the reality of that state. The other state is my normal, familiar self—talkative, busy, happy, enthusiastic, and energetic.

The problem is the transition between these two states. Going from normal to chemo state happens pretty naturally and quickly. I don't feel myself getting depressed or upset. But moving from chemo state back to normal, I experience the worst psychological part of this journey so far. While it's difficult to articulate, with each round, it takes more days to move back into wanting to talk with people, be busy with things, and get back to living. This round, I felt physically better by Friday, but it was Monday before I fully embraced leaving the house.

By about Saturday, five days after the treatment, I start to realize what's going on, but it's impossible for me to change the way I feel. It may just be a matter of the time it takes for the drugs to wear off. Since chemo is cumulative, it takes more days each round for me to recover back to my regular personality. The whole time I'm watching myself and thinking, *You should call so-and-so to get caught up* or *You should start checking e-mail* or *The house won't clean itself*—but it's impossible for me to get anything done. And it's not because I'm too fatigued or physically ill; it's just that my mind is still sort of blank, and I don't want to be connected to anyone or anything. I want to be left alone. Perhaps this awareness of the process will help me deal with the next round.

Tonight, Vivian and I went ice-skating for the first time this winter. It was lovely. That's another bonus of having kids—without her, I never would have gone out on the rink tonight! I'm happy to be feeling very much myself tonight. It's good to be back.

Graduation Day!
Friday, December 14, 2007, 7:47 a.m.

Graduation day! Yesterday, I graduated from physical therapy. It's great to have that item crossed off my list. My right arm is in the clear now, but I still need to be careful of developing lymphedema. The short list of preventive measures includes maintaining my nails perfectly; being very careful of my skin care; always wearing sunscreen to prevent burns and insect repellent to avoid bug bites; moving my arm around when on an airplane or during a long car ride; avoiding right-arm accidental cuts, blood draws, needle pokes, and blood-pressure checks; staying away from exercise that heats me too much, hot tubs, saunas, and deep-tissue massage on the right side of my back and arm. Other than those things, I'm footloose and fancy-free.

I went to the gym again yesterday. It was a much better experience this time. I had a moderate workout, including cardio and weights. It's helping my mood and energy level quite a bit. I hope to get there tomorrow too, which would be the most workouts in one single week AD (after diagnosis). It feels very normal to be back at the gym, in the same way it feels so normal to be at the office. I'm also starting to believe that while my health isn't perfect, when I'm at the gym, I'm actively doing something to improve it.

Jackson is calling me now. Gotta run.

Feeling Better
Monday, December 17, 2007, 7:46 a.m.

This weekend was great. It seems impossible, but I kept forgetting about cancer. It was helpful to have something to look forward to at every moment like baking cookies with Vivian and holiday shopping with Wade while the kids were with a babysitter. I'm really looking forward to Christmas.

Sleep has been easy to find lately. I've been falling asleep with Vivian after reading to her around 8:30 p.m., and staying asleep until 6:30 a.m. I wonder if needing so much sleep is a function of the cumulative nature of the chemo. Guess I'll find out with my next round the day after Christmas.

I have to visit the clinic for a blood draw today, but I'm not worried about it yet. My white count was low last time, as was my red count, so if they aren't up by today, I'll be in for more medication to boost them. I feel so much better than I did last week. It seems like my levels must be doing better, but I won't know for sure until after my labs. Last night, we had to cancel dinner with Jackson's godparents because his godfather had a cold. It was a drag, but I just can't risk getting sick now.

Beautiful Dream

Tuesday, December 18, 2007, 7:07 a.m.

My mom is so proud of her Swedish heritage and several years ago found an opportunity for Vivian to participate in a Swedish folk dance troupe. The dancing and costumes are adorable. Part of the reason I had such a great weekend was something that happened on Friday night at Vivian's performance. One of her fellow folk dancers recently lost his mother to ovarian cancer. I had a chance to talk with the dad about his wife's journey. He gave me some really good advice for dealing with cancer and young children. His wife had been terminal for quite some time. He told me they had a saying: "Live each day like you'll live forever." Really struck a chord.

Last night, I dreamed our family had to leave Minnesota for Arizona. I was upset because I had to leave some things behind, things I'd never get back. Wade took the journey with the kids, but I had to travel alone. Once I arrived by plane, it was a long, long car ride to the apartment we rented sight unseen. Once I got there, I walked a long way from the entrance of the building to our apartment. I passed things along the way: a great game room, a nice restaurant, a bar, a lecture hall, an exercise room. Once I got to the apartment, a guy took me on a tour of the place. It was beautiful, fully furnished, and huge. The view out the living room window was amazing, a stunning Arizona landscape. The only catch? A fleet of construction trucks was tearing up the space just outside our apartment. It was temporary, but really noisy and disruptive.

The chemo is that fleet of powerful, dangerous, noisy trucks, tearing up my life. And I have to take the journey alone. I get it.

Perspective Shift
Saturday, December 22, 2007, 4:32 p.m.

With Christmas just around the corner, somehow I've been able to forget all about chemo coming up on December 26. While I know it's coming, I haven't been dreading it like I normally do. Christmas Eve and Christmas Day are so full of activity that it's hard to think past those two busy days. Plus, I'm looking forward to seeing the kids open their gifts.

I recently experienced a big shift of perspective on how I view people with illness or disability. I saw a woman in a wheelchair at the shopping mall. She was with a friend and had her hair and makeup done. She obviously cared about how she looked. She had tchotchkes on her chair and seemed happy to be hanging out with her friend. I used to see people with disabilities and think, *I'm so grateful for my health.* But now I see people with disabilities and think, *There's a person living life, getting out and about even though it's not easy. She must have some interesting stories to tell.* I admire them—they've weathered some storms and lived to tell about it.

During my last round of chemo, I started thinking about shut-ins, which is basically what I am for the four or five days I don't leave my bedroom after a chemo treatment. While I don't want to get out during those days, I'd go mad looking at the same four walls year after year. I wonder how shut-ins feel when visitors come around.

We took our best outing of the season on Thursday night. One of my clients asked if our family could join him at the Holidazzle parade. For those of you outside Minnesota, Holidazzle is something that can only happen here. It's a holiday parade that goes through downtown Minneapolis. All the floats and costumes are covered in Christmas lights. It's amazing! My client has a retired city bus totally covered in Christmas lights called the Twinkle Bus, and he invited us to ride in it. Vivian was in her element. Most of the route, she stood near the bus driver, singing "Feliz Navidad" and shouting, "Merry Christmas!" out the open window. Jack also waved to people out the bus window. It was something we'll always remember.

Wade and I have decided to eat with abandon for the holidays, and we've been enjoying cookies and candy like crazy. We'll worry about the consequences after the first of the year!

Close Call

Tuesday, December 25, 2007, 11:30 p.m.

I'm not sure where to begin. In past years, I'd spend so much time projecting what Christmas Eve or Christmas Day should be like that I'd often feel disappointed. This year, I found myself enjoying each moment and each new surprise as it passed.

One of the blessings of the last three months (it's been three months and one day since my surgery!) is that I've communicated with so many people I'd lost touch with—and I'm so much closer to my friends than I was before. Hearing their Christmas greetings was even more meaningful this year.

Having our financial worries relieved for the short term by the pottery sale also made Christmas more enjoyable this year. While we're still not rich, at least we have my medical expenses covered for next year, and we made up the equivalent of about a weeks' worth of the work that Wade and I missed. We're feeling much more relaxed living two paychecks ahead, rather than paycheck to paycheck.

Vivian was so patient teaching Jackson how to open his gifts. She was also generous, up to a point, with sharing her new toys with her little brother. Dr. Rocko, our big orange cat, even tolerated the Christmas ribbon I tied around his neck for a good fifteen minutes before I felt sorry for him and removed it. Savannah, our black Lab–Doberman mix, and our young white cat, Cedric, didn't have to endure any ribbons. We have yet to hold hands and sing "Oh Christmas Tree" encircling the tree as Vivian suggested earlier in the season, but just thinking about it has created a lovely memory for me.

Then, this morning, we were driving in the fresh snow. As I drove Wade and the kids to my cousin's house, I started to merge onto the freeway. I was about to comment to Wade that it seemed like one of those times when there could be hidden patches of ice. Before I could voice that thought, as I accelerated and turned the wheel to merge onto the freeway, my car started to spin out of control.

I read the obituaries this morning (which I never do) and came across a thirty-nine-old woman who'd lost control of her car. "Don't hit the brakes," Wade calmly reminded me. I must have turned the steering wheel the correct direction, because after spinning clockwise and then counterclockwise, we stopped. We came within inches of hitting the median, and the other cars were able to stop in time before hitting us—though one almost couldn't before she slipped past us. My car came to a stop within a few feet of the Mississippi River Bridge. Vivian was really shaken up.

After that adrenaline rush, I was thinking about that song from the musical *Rent*, "Seasons of Love," that asks:

525,600 minutes, 525,000 moments so dear. 525,600 minutes— how do you measure, measure a year? In daylights, in sunsets, in midnights, in cups of coffee. In inches, in miles, in laughter, in strife . . . . In truths that she learned, or in times that he cried. In bridges he burned, or the way that she died. It's time now to sing out, tho the story never ends. Let's celebrate, remember a year in the life of friends. Remember the love! Measure in love. Seasons of love.

The love Wade shows me continues to amaze. Despite so many scars, a bald head, an often grumpy attitude, a demanding voice, and once-identical twins (wink) that now look more like fraternal twins, he still continues to sincerely find me attractive and often shows me in inappropriate ways.

The baby that we remember on Christmas Day is alive and well in my world tonight. May you find peace in your heart for many of the 525,600 minutes in the new year and in all the years you experience on this sometimes confusing, often lovely path we journey together.

More IV Fluids

Thursday, January 3, 2008, 7:26 p.m.

The chemo was OK. It made me way more fatigued this time, but no nausea. The only smell problems I experienced were with chemicals, not food odors. I even had to steer clear of strongly scented soaps and household cleaners. I also started experiencing some weird aversions. One of the IV drugs I get, Adriamycin, is bright red, like Tropical Punch Kool-Aid. Now I find myself unable to drink anything red.

Just as I started feeling more energy around New Year's Eve, my energy tanked again on New Year's Day. By the next day, I was back in the clinic getting IV fluids. My doctor concluded that I have the flu. I went back to the clinic again today for another two liters of fluids and was awake all afternoon, which was a big improvement. I need to get another liter of fluids tomorrow. Maybe I'll be back to work tomorrow afternoon? My fever is down to 99.2, so hopefully it will be gone tomorrow. Through all these days when I need to be in the clinic, I'm even more appreciative that my mom is able to watch Jackson during the day and meet Vivian at school in the afternoon. Her ability to keep the kids safe and happy is so important.

This chemo treatment, without something tangible coming up (like a Minnesota Wild game or Christmas) to look forward to, I find myself having more dark thoughts than I have in the past. Just the idea of going back out into the world for work, book group, or a party seems too overwhelming to even consider. The cold, cloudy, gray weather may be contributing to that.

The Last in Line
Sunday, January 6, 2008, 7:33 p.m.

The light at the end of the tunnel is becoming visible. Only two more chemos left. I'm so glad this treatment is finite—with a specific number prescribed from the very start. It seems much easier than dealing with something ongoing without a clear end date. After being through four treatments, at least I know what to expect.

On Friday after getting fluids at the clinic, I went to the office for the afternoon. It was so great to be there. It's funny that just a few days earlier, I felt as if I'd never be strong enough to make it back to work or go anywhere.

Even though I had to drag myself to church this morning, it was good to get out of the house. Once again, Vivian sang in the children's choir and looked so beautiful in her choir robe. I still have a cough and stuffed-up nose, so I sat toward the back of the church. Although I wasn't in the last row, something I've never experienced happened. When I got to the Communion rail, I realized I'd be the last person to take Communion. The Episcopal church still uses a common cup, so as I took the wine, I imagined all the power, strength, and hope of the entire congregation who had drunk from that same cup minutes earlier, infusing me.

When I was sitting in church, I felt so hot. I had to take off my sweater and wear just my camisole while seated. I wondered if my fever was back, but when I got home, I had no fever. Now I think it may have been hot flashes. My oncologist mentioned the chemo would force me into menopause. He said it's time to start reading about it, so I know what to expect.

The kids are ready for bed, so I'll read to Vivian now. We've been enjoying some great times lately, just the two of us.

Missing Hair

Tuesday, January 8, 2008, 11:41 p.m.

Wow. It's way past my bedtime. Had a great time at book group tonight and then hanging out with Wade after I got home. Wade learned something funny about Jackson tonight—he's deathly afraid of Mylar balloons. The latex ones, he loves, but their safer cousins give him nightmares. He actually woke from a nightmare tonight saying, "Balloon." Poor little man. He's twenty-one months old now, and Vivian turns seven in a few days.

Sometimes Vivian will say, "Mom, I wish you had hair." And I'll say, "Me too." Lately, I've been missing my old hair. I look forward to growing it again. When I first lost it, I didn't think it was such a big deal, considering the alternative. But now I'm burned out on the wig-scarf-bandana scene.

One woman at my church is about two months ahead of me in her treatment; she's done with chemo and partway through radiation. She's been wearing scarves the whole time. On Sunday, I noticed a little bit of hair growing at the edge of her scarf, and she happily reported that, yes, it's coming back. Like a crocus in the snow, her little bit of hair gave me so much hope.

In just one month, I'll be due for my last chemo session. It's exciting to think that I'm so close to being done with the worst of this treatment. Radiation will be a drag because I'll have to go to the clinic five days a week, but the side effects are minor, so I won't have to miss work. After missing so much work—and hating missing it—I've come to suspect that I'll be one of those people who never retires. You know the newspaper articles about the little old man who's ninety but still goes to his office every day? That will totally be me. Too much leisure time makes me nervous. I need to feel like I have some purpose to my life.

On the other hand . . . I'm learning to go slow. Last night, I just lay on the couch while Jackson played with his oversized toddler-safe Lego blocks. He didn't need me, so I just watched him put his blocks together. Four months ago, I probably would have stood up to look for something productive to do. Instead, I got to watch my cute little man.

Bone Pain Fears

Saturday, January 12, 2008, 10:01 p.m.

Yesterday was Vivian's seventh birthday. We had her party at our house. She had so much fun. I love to tell her about the first time I saw her— how beautiful she looked and how I told her I'd love her forever. Wade always brags to her that he was the first person ever to hold her (the doctor let him catch her at the last minute). Vivian loves to hear these stories, and her birthday is a great excuse to tell them. The day before her party, she asked if I'd be wearing my wig (often I just wear a hat or nothing in the evening, after wearing a wig all day), and when I told her I would wear my wig, she said, "Whew!"

The thing I'm dreading most about my final rounds of chemo is a shot I get the day after to boost my white count. One of the side effects is bone pain. After receiving this shot the first few times, my hips hurt a little bit. This last round, the pain ran down my legs and up my spine. If muscles hurt, generally movement will bring some relief, but movement makes the bone pain worse. Even sitting still, the pain from this medication is on the same level as giving birth—which I know because I didn't take pain meds during childbirth with either kid. I'm worried that these final rounds of chemo and the day-after white-count booster shot will cause unbearable pain.

Genetic Test Anxiety

Wednesday, January 16, 2008, 8:55 p.m.

Cancer has educated me about health insurance. With our existing policy, I'll pay the full amount for everything until I hit my $3,000 out-of-pocket maximum, and then insurance will kick in at 100 percent. A painful example of the plan in action: I went to pick up my antinausea drugs at the pharmacy this morning and paid $623. They're worth every penny, but it *freaked* me out. I didn't have enough in our checking account . . . so the credit card came to the rescue.

My oncologist, Dr. Anderson, is pushing me to get a genetic test to determine if I carry the breast cancer (BRCA1 or BRCA2) genetic mutation. Having this genetic information will help guide my post-radiation treatment. Today, I attended a breast cancer conference and saw a presentation on the importance of genetic testing. If I test negative for the gene, my chances for getting breast cancer again increase just 1 percent every year I live. If I test positive for the gene, my chances of getting another breast cancer jump immediately to 60 percent. A positive result would make me seriously consider a double mastectomy and surgical removal of the ovaries, because there's a proven relationship between breast and ovarian cancer.

The test should also help the kids plan their futures. If I test positive, they'll each have a 50 percent chance of having the same genetic mutation. Vivian will be eligible for an annual mammogram and MRI (starting at age twenty-five), regardless of her genetic status due to my relatively young age at the time of diagnosis. There are some pretty noninvasive ways of lowering her chances for breast cancer if she has the mutation.

I was worried my health insurance provider could dump me if I tested positive and that I'd have trouble finding new insurance if I was kicked off my existing insurance. The geneticist explained that under the Health Insurance Portability and Accountability Act (HIPAA), it's illegal to discriminate based on genes. As she put it, the gene is not the disease. So my insurance should be secure.

For chemo tomorrow, I'm feeling pretty good. The sense of dread hasn't been there this time. I'm looking forward to it in a weird way, just knowing that it's the second to last. Bring it on.

The prechemo steroids are keeping me up tonight; I can see why athletes love 'em. They give me so much energy I can clean the entire house and be cheerful while I'm doing it.

I've started having more "chemo brain," which presents as being spacey. I don't remember what I'm doing, I forget things, I have a difficult time concentrating. I've always been a huge note-taker and list maker, so those habits have been helping out, but it's scary to think how much of my job depends on me remembering something from a conversation, knowing a deadline, completing all the steps in a task. Even typing is less efficient, because I make more mistakes. At least it's temporary.

I guess this is good-bye for a while. I'll write again when I step out of the fog. Love to you all until then!

P.S. Poor Wade is feeling very neglected lately. Please send your prayers and give him hugs and gifts when you see him!

Chemo Sucks

Wednesday, January 23, 2008, 8:39 a.m.

Have I mentioned that chemo SUCKS?! It really is terrible. The nausea and smell sensitivity came roaring back, but I didn't get sick or dehydrated. I have energy to be awake but not enough energy to actually do anything. It's an awful limbo. The four walls of the bedroom, even the view out the window, bore me so much I can't stand it.

During the last two rounds of chemo, I've dug into my memories. I'll fixate on a time and place, like my college dorm room. I'll explore the place in detail, like a ghost traveling through the space. It's like that time before you leave a job—after you've quit, but you're still around for the last two weeks to wrap things up. People start asking who can have your stapler. Nobody wants to invest in too much conversation because you'll be gone, and so you start traveling through space more quietly. That's what I've done in my mind the last few days.

Marathon Obstacle Course

Sunday, January 27, 2008, 12:05 a.m.

On Wednesday, I went to work because I was feeling so much better. I surrounded myself with people who'd make me feel better, and I even made it to the gym.

The last time I went in for a Neulasta shot—the white-blood-cell booster—Wade asked if there's anything other than Tylenol I could take for the bone pain it causes. They sent me home with a prescription for Vicodin.

That same day, I mentioned to a coworker that I was feeling so great and that I didn't think I'd need the Vicodin. I forgot to knock on wood. Three hours later, I got into my car, and stabbing pain shot through my hips and up into my spine. Damn. I crawled into bed with a heating pad and thanked the good Lord for my new drug.

In other news, I've realized something important about self-pity. It's OK to catalog the things I miss from my old life. It's not easy to be in a dark place, but the mourning process requires a dark place sometimes. That night as I lay in bed after taking the Vicodin, afraid to move for fear of pain, I let myself remember all the things I used to have that I'll never have again. I let myself cry about what a long marathon this is becoming. Today, someone reminded me this journey is a marathon *and* an obstacle course—at the twenty-third mile, I've been forced to start jumping hurdles while I run.

On Thursday, I woke up afraid to move. I lay in bed all morning, not even getting up for the bathroom. Each time the medication wore off, the pain crept back. Stabbing pain across my hips, down my legs, up my spine, and a new pain in my chest. It felt like something was sitting on my chest, and it hurt to take a deep breath. My hips and back hurt as much as they did when I was in pre-childbirth labor (sans drugs, remember?) At 11:00 a.m., I talked to my nurse, who told me to get out of bed and start moving my joints. That helped a little, though the pain lasted all day. She also said I could negotiate about the white-count booster shot after my final round of chemo with Dr. Anderson. Then, hopefully, this pain will vanish forever.

On Friday, I felt better physically but somehow staying in bed all day Thursday wore me out—if that even makes sense. I knew I couldn't just eat Vicodin all day, but I didn't want to go to work. Would you call that lazy? I felt lazy, so I went to work. And it helped to get moving and focus on something positive.

I was supposed to go to the clinic after work, but just the thought made me sick to my stomach, so I skipped. This is the first week since September 14 that I haven't had at least one doctor's appointment! AWOL, and loving every minute of it.

Tonight, we went to my company party, and I wore my "Bobalicious" wig for the first time. A little more than flirty, Bobalicious loves to stay out late and tell tall tales the next morning but can still pass as a churchgoer when necessary. To go with my flirtier wig, I wore more makeup than usual, and Vivian was quite appalled. She said I looked like a Bratz doll—the dolls we've banned in our house because they're even more hooker-like than Barbie. Plus, the name Bratz implies bad behavior. Barbie at least pretends to be a veterinarian or schoolteacher. Bratz dolls admit they're just groupies. It was pretty funny to have my seven-year-old disapprove of my makeup based on the appearance of the dolls that I disapprove of because of their makeup. Can't wait 'til she's a teen!

Hanging on to Eyelashes
Tuesday, January 29, 2008, 9:48 p.m.

Turns out I misunderstood Vivian when I thought she was scolding me for looking like a Bratz doll. On Sunday morning, I was about to leave the house, and she said, "Mommy, you should wear the makeup you wore last night. You looked so good!" Guess I'll have to glam it up more often.

I have been wearing my Bobalicious wig pretty much nonstop because I'm bored with Anne. Now that it's been several months without hair, I just feel like none of the wigs, scarves, hats, or even bald head are really me. I'm ready for real hair again. It will take years for it to be as long as it was, but it will be worth the wait. My eyebrows and eyelashes are so thin now that there's not much left to lose. One survivor warned me that while her hair started growing back three weeks after her final chemo, her eyebrows and eyelashes only started growing back two weeks after that. I'm holding on to each eyelash and eyebrow hair as long as possible.

The Final Countdown

Monday, February 4, 2008, 9:09 p.m.

Three days and counting until my final chemo. While I'm not dreading it, I am wondering how many days it will take to recover. With each round, it has taken a little bit longer to feel better. I've been sleeping so much, still ten to eleven hours per night. I really miss those two or three evening hours I used to have after the kids were asleep to get things done around the house.

Did I mention that I'm anemic? About a month ago, Dr. Anderson gave me the expected news. He prescribed iron pills, which I rarely remember to take. For about a week now, I've been much better about taking them, and that has been increasing my energy level.

The increased energy facilitated ice-skating the other night. All the way around the rink, Vivian sang a song to the tune of "Joy to the World":

> *Joy to the world, Barney's dead!*
> *We barbecued his head!*
> *Don't worry 'bout his body.*
> *We used it for karate.*

Oh, the things they learn in first grade these days. I know I shouldn't laugh, but it does crack me up. I've never been a big fan of that purple blob.

My final treatment is also my final descent into the chemo underworld, or wherever it is I go. The sermon at church on Sunday mentioned thin places—places where the boundaries are blurred between heaven and earth, the spirit world and the human world. The mountaintop where Jesus went to meditate and pray was the context for the discussion of thin places. I realized it's a thin place I go to after chemo. While it's difficult to articulate, I learn things when I'm there. I've learned the most important things are love and kindness and that the only things we get to keep are the things we've given away. For this final chemo, while I don't want to experience the tummy trouble or total exhaustion, it's my last chance to experience this type of thin place. I wonder what I'll learn.

Wade and Vivian have been telling me that I have blonde peach fuzz on my head, and yesterday at the gym I noticed it in the mirror. If it's blonde or white, I'm not sure, but it will be fun to see if it sticks around after this final round. My eyebrows and eyelashes are almost gone. Both can be counted in single digits! I'm adding pencil to my remaining eyebrows, and nobody seems to notice they're mostly fake. At least nobody has the guts to mention it to me.

Prechemo Pig-Out
Wednesday, February 6, 2008, 8:54 p.m.

Had my prechemo pig-out this evening. Almost a whole Chipotle burrito with chips and guacamole, followed by five Dove dark chocolate squares. For my bedtime snack, I have nutritionally devoid snack toast waiting on the kitchen counter. In case you don't know, it's prepackaged dried white toast with cinnamon sugar on top. I always add a ton of butter to it. When we first met, Wade thought it was totally gross and something only a Swede could eat (by the way, he's part Swedish too), but now he loves it.

Lately, I've been feeling less and less attractive. It takes more and more makeup to look halfway normal. But I got a boost at Chipotle. (Here's where I wish Wade didn't read this blog. Maybe he'll miss this entry.) The one flirty guy there flirted with me again tonight. It's been a long time since I've had a second look from a guy, so that was fun. He's always flirting with everyone—but still, I'll take flirting from anyone these days. When I mentioned that the plain rice and cheese tacos were for my kids, he said, "You don't look like you have any kids," which is totally untrue, but still, the flattery was appreciated.

My peach fuzz seems to be growing daily. I'm so excited to have hair again; it will make me feel so much better about how I look. While it's growing back, I'll start out with a boy-cut style because I'll have no choice. I've always thought women with boy cuts and pixies are so gutsy and adorable, but I've never had the nerve to try one of those styles. It will be interesting to see how I look with hair so short.

I'm on the 'roids again, so I've been really energetic (and kind of sweaty) today. Each chemo cycle, I take steroids the day before and the day after the treatment. I'll have a few pills left over after tomorrow, and it will indeed be tempting in the future to take them when I need a little boost. Knowing me, I'll be a good girl and just dispose of pills in the most environmentally friendly manner.

It's a good thing I have extra energy today, because getting ready for chemo is much like the day before leaving on vacation. I need to get my work all wrapped up, give instructions to my backup at the office, tidy my desk, put my e-mail on autoreply, record an out-of-office voice mail message, get the house somewhat clean, make sure I have a week's worth of clean clothes, and get the bills paid. This list makes me thankful for the steroids.

I'm excited that this is my last chemo (knock on wood), but I'm still dreading it. One of my main signs of stress is memory loss. Yesterday, I couldn't remember numbers I normally keep in my head for work. I also forgot the names of people I've known for a long time. The knowledge that I'll be even sicker after this round of chemo is clearly causing quite a bit of stress.

Vivian is so happy it's my final chemo. I love that she keeps close track of what's going on with me. She's been touching the peach fuzz on my head and trying to figure out how quickly my hair will grow. She wants me to grow it long again right away so she can braid, curl, and style it like she used to when I had long hair.

I've been totally healthy my whole life—until, at age thirty-one, I had my thyroid removed; at age thirty-four, I had bunion surgery on my right foot; and at thirty-eight, breast cancer. All these things typically strike women in their sixties, seventies, or eighties. Each has made me feel like an old woman trapped in a young woman's body. Yesterday, I realized that because I've had all these old-lady ailments already, that when I'm an actual old woman, I'll be healthy as a horse and still driving my car at ninety-five. (Are you reading this, God?) Hopefully, we'll have hovercrafts by then so I can really terrify those young whippersnappers out on the skies.

Still Exhausted

Wednesday, February 13, 2008, 6:58 p.m.

A week after chemo. Still exhausted. I keep thinking a big boost of energy is just around the corner, but I have yet to find it. On Monday, I was ready for an outing, so Wade and I walked the full city block to Vivian's school for her first-grade program. It was a half-hour history presentation with singing. I was so excited to be out that I thought we could go shopping afterward, but I was way too wiped out after the program for any shopping. The presentation wasn't exhausting, but I hadn't planned on seeing a bunch of parents at the event, all wanting to know how I was feeling. It was overwhelming to talk with so many people when I still felt off-kilter.

Today, I've gone out several times with Jackson (it's finally twenty degrees and warm enough to get out). We walked around the block with Vivian's rolling backpack, which Jackson loves to pull behind him. It must have appeared to the neighbors like Jackson's parent-aided runaway attempt. Now he's walking around the dining room table with his bubble mower, sans bubbles.

My brain still isn't functioning at 100 percent. Today, I called my neighbor, and as I left a message, I couldn't quite come up with my phone number. It's difficult to think fast right now. I'm looking forward to the full return of my brain.

We haven't marked this last round of chemo with any kind of party just yet. The nurses at the clinic wanted to have a celebration, but I was feeling so down and so sick by the time we left that I waved it off. I'm not quite feeling chemo is over, because I'm still queasy, mostly from outdoor smells like diesel fuel. And as a nurse put it, nausea and hunger are very close together. Today, I've been like a newborn, feeling starving, and needing to eat every two hours.

On Sunday, my cousin Melissa and her husband, Uri, are hosting an end-of-chemo dinner. Also joining will be my mom, my cousin Sunny, her husband, Mike, my cousin Mike, his wife, Ruth, plus some of my cousins' kids. I'm looking forward to that as my official celebration, eating good food, and relaxing with family.

I still fear bone pain. It hasn't manifested yet, but last night I was so scared that I took Vicodin in the middle of the night before I even needed it. The fear of pain can be just as troubling as the pain itself.

I asked Dr. Anderson to forgo the final white-count booster shot, but he said no way. The last time he let someone skip a final shot, the person ended up in the hospital with a life-threatening infection. I said no thanks to that. I'll take the pain instead.

As for going to some faraway place, a thin place, or spiritual journey . . . well, it just didn't happen this time. My mind stayed pretty much in the moment most of the time. It was nice to feel somewhat intact.

Tomorrow is the five-month anniversary of my diagnosis. It's hard to believe it's been that long and that short of a time. For some reason, these anniversaries seem important to remember—as a way to contemplate how much things have changed and how much they've stayed the same.

Today, Jackson slept on my chest, and I just hung out letting him sleep for over an hour. Five months ago, I never would have done that. I used to be moving all the time. Wade would implore me each evening to join him to watch TV and "stop milling about" the house. Will I be able to maintain this ability to just hang out? Probably not, because if I'd have had the energy today, I'm sure I would have jumped up after ten minutes and started the laundry. I think the ability to rest will stick with me at least enough to notice what's going on in the moment and enjoy it.

Speaking of rest, it's time to start getting the kids ready for bed. I might not even stay up past their bedtimes tonight.

Ice Cream Social in the Sky

Saturday, February 16, 2008, 4:51 p.m.

Thursday night, the bone pain started, so I spent two days with my old buddy Vicodin. Now the pain has passed, and I feel great. I did a good job of staying on top of the medication by taking it on time, so I never had to stay in bed with a heating pad. Pain management is a science and an art.

I'm still low energy. I fall asleep by 8:30 p.m. and sleep as late as possible, usually until 6:00 a.m. During the day, I need to sit or lie down a couple of times just to take a break. A major side effect of the radiation I'll start in two weeks is fatigue, but I can live with being exhausted on a daily basis as long as I don't have to spend day after day in bed.

On Valentine's Day, I helped with Vivian's class party. It's cute how excited kids get when they can eat candy at school. Poor Vivian got really sick last night and threw up a few times. Wade, as usual, was the one on hazmat duty. He's so sweet; he said he doesn't mind because whatever he's cleaning up, he's had to clean something worse in the past. Vivian went to bed early and woke up feeling just fine this morning. So far, she's having a great day. It's over thirty degrees outside, so it's been fun to get outdoors again.

Lately, I've been wishing that Wade would keep a journal. I know that it's been difficult for him, but now that I'm starting to feel better, I wish that I could know more what it's been like for him all this time. He's been spending some time doing self-care (having a few beers with the boys, working in his art studio), so his mood has been much better the last few weeks. He's had to endure so much during this time. I'm glad he can relax a little bit.

Part of why I'm thinking about journals is because after retiring as a nurse, my cute little mom took on the huge project of learning Swedish to translate her grandfather's memoir. He came to the United States from Sweden in the 1890s and wrote a comprehensive account of all the places he'd worked across the upper Midwest. He also wrote about family life both in Sweden and America. My mom finally completed the project, and she's been sharing some of the stories, photos, and documents with me. I'm so grateful that she translated these precious documents. She's been the official historian in several nursing organizations she's belonged to, and I'm glad she's using those skills to capture our family history.

On Thursday night, my mom shared the letter my great-grandmother Hulda wrote as she was dying in the hospital in 1930. The letter was addressed to her pet name for her husband—"My little Gust," short for August. She writes that she felt it was just time to finally go, but she worried about the expense it would cause. She apologized for her poor handwriting and understated the obvious by writing, "I don't have my eyeglasses with me. I'm feeling anxious and a little sad." She implored Gust to be nice to his granddaughter (Illeane, my aunt) and keep his faith in God so he could look forward to them being together in heaven. It was so sweet and amazing that she was relatively calm even as she saw death just around the corner. To be "a little sad" is such an understatement. But in the context of her faith, it makes sense. In his memoir, my great-grandfather writes that his saddest day was when his Hulda died, but that he knew the Lord was keeping her in his strong arms until they could be together again.

I thought of these things as I drifted off to sleep Thursday night. I thought about my version of heaven and how wonderful it will be to meet these kind and stoic great-grandparents who died before I was born. I thought about meeting other ancestors from way back and later, meeting future descendants and my hopefully long-lived friends. Heaven in my imagination has always been a beautiful, sunny, outdoor space, peaceful, with lots of people and conversation to enjoy—like an ice-cream social in a park. Nobody really knows what happens after we die, so why not imagine something wonderful? Plus, life is better with a really big party to look forward to after it's all over. Thinking about all of this, I felt joy. I started to realize: I'm back. I don't mean just back to myself after this round of chemo. Some of the innocence, trust, and happiness that I lost through this experience are finally coming back. It was the happiest that I've felt in a long time.

Nose Hair

Wednesday, February 20, 2008, 9:06 p.m.

What kind of self-respecting woman wishes for, longs for, nose hair? I think you know the answer. For the past few weeks, my nose has been constantly running. I've had to carry a Kleenex everywhere I go. Without nose hair, there's nothing to stop the running. Count it as one more thing to look forward to in the upcoming weeks. Oh, nose hair, I never thought I'd miss you!

In other news, I'm still tired, still going to bed early. My skin is drier than it's ever been. That's one of the side effects I didn't experience until the last few weeks of chemo. I've been slopping on the moisturizer like mad, and it helps, but within hours, my skin dries out again. I realize now why my doctor scheduled only six rounds of chemo—another round feels like it would kill me or at least do permanent damage.

The hustle and bustle of work is refreshing after spending so much time resting. I'm noticing that being really busy for the last few days has me living on a much more surface, less reflective level. I don't think it's a bad thing; I've been happy to get a ton of things done.

I've been cleaning and organizing the house, and I've started caring about my appearance again. With the first chemo, I had to quit using whitening toothpaste, due to the smell, and now I'm back on it. Before all of this, I religiously flossed daily (yes, I'm one of those people) but had to give it up for lack of energy. Now I'm back on the floss. I also started doing some at-home minifacials. But with my skin so dry, I accidentally irritated the skin on my nose. So in my efforts to look better, I ended up looking more like Rudolph the Red-Nosed Reindeer than someone who had just gotten a facial. Oh well.

The end-of-chemo celebration dinner at Melissa and Uri's house on Sunday was lovely. The food was great, and I was given a bouquet of roses, snapdragons, and a hydrangea plant. My mom seemed happy to celebrate that the worst of the treatments are behind us. As the party wrapped up, I really did feel like we had marked the end of the chemo phase of treatment. Those rituals and celebrations are important. I'm so glad Melissa and Uri thought of having that dinner for me.

Weekly Blood Draw
Thursday, February 21, 2008, 6:01 p.m.

This afternoon, I went to my clinic for a weekly blood draw. For the first time in months, I didn't get sick to my stomach an hour before the appointment. Going to the clinic directly from work, wearing my brown tweed suit and work ID on its lanyard, I pretended I was just going to a work appointment. It was late in the day, so the place was deserted, which was also nice. Best of all, I know I don't ever have to return there for chemo.

The blood draw itself still creates a visceral reaction. The port they use for the draw is positioned between my left breast and left collarbone. Its tube goes into my jugular vein and then directly into my heart. When they inject saline to flush the port, it makes for a really awful taste in my mouth. Normally, I remember to grab a piece of candy first, but I forgot today. Luckily, the nurse gave me a Jolly Rancher as the yucky taste started. Having that taste (even with the candy, it's still there) in my mouth makes me feel a bit gross for a few hours afterward.

It cracks me up how much candy is at the oncology clinic. On nearly every horizontal surface, there's a bowl of candy. Mostly cheap hard candy, along with some Tootsie Rolls. Never good chocolate, but I used to think the message was, "Sucks that you have cancer, but at least you can have some candy while you wait for your appointment." But now I realize it's more likely intended for people with a port to avoid that icky taste after a blood draw.

Poor Wade is sick today. He still went to work, and now he's with Jackson and Vivian at the school talent show. It's a two-and-a-half-hour ordeal that Vivian cried her way into convincing Wade to attend. Our kids aren't even performing. I'm sure it won't be long, though, before Vivian's up there on stage, and we're all sitting rapt in the audience for hours on end.

With the rest of the family out of the house, I have time to myself before I leave for book group. We're going to celebrate the end of my chemo, another member's job promotion, and the addition of a new person to our group. So while it's normally pop and wine, tonight it's champagne and sparkling fruit juice. But I'd better load the dishwasher before I leave.

You Can't Return

Tuesday, February 26, 2008, 9:59 p.m.

I've been back to work for a week. I really feel as if life is getting back to normal. But the words of my surgeon keep haunting me. He said you can never really return to life before cancer. It's true. I'm questioning everything. During my last chemo, I made a long list of things I'd like to do. Most aren't costly or time consuming; they mainly involve reconnecting with friends and nature. The thing I learned in those thin places during chemo was that the most important things are kindness and love. I learned that the only things we get to keep are those we give away. So I'm examining how I can best serve those around me. I hope writing this narrative is one way to help others.

Physically, I'm feeling well, but I'm disappointed in how much sleep I still require. For the most part, I fall asleep beside Vivian after we finish her bedtime reading, get up and go to bed, and sleep until 7:00 a.m. According to the mirror, I have bags under my eyes; those are new. Tonight, I'm up way past my bedtime, and I'm sure to be sorry in the morning.

My meeting with the radiation oncologist is in two days. I wasn't worried about radiation, but now I'm getting nervous. Mostly, it's thinking about the possible burns. My understanding is that careful skin care will prevent problems, and I hope that's true. My skin has become increasingly dry even though chemo has ended. It looks thinner and older all the time, so I'm worried that my skin isn't in great shape for radiation.

The warmer (thirty-five degrees!) weather has been wonderful for the soul. Vivian and I have taken a couple of long walks. I love spending time with that little lady. She's been really fantastic during this rough time. The other day before book group, she asked, "Are you sure you'll be feeling well enough to go?" I was happy to remind her that I won't be feeling sick anymore, unless I get the flu. I know that Vivian gets much of her caring attitude from my mom, who's passing down her sweetness and concern for others to Vivian.

At the time of my diagnosis, we were within a week of signing a new mortgage to put a second story on our house. For several years, we've been planning with my mom to build three bedrooms and a bath upstairs so we could convert the two downstairs bedrooms and downstairs bathroom into a mother-in-law apartment for her. She's in great health but doesn't need her big house anymore. And we'd like for her to be closer to us, which she'd like too because she's here so often helping with the kids. The plan was to make a kitchenette in her apartment so she could have breakfast and lunch on her own and then join us for dinner each evening. We postponed the plan so I could recover in peace without workmen tromping through the house. Now, we're in the process of refinalizing our plans so we can start on the construction this spring.

Snow Falling on a Bare Head
Thursday, February 28, 2008, 10:13 p.m.

Today brought lots of good news, but it didn't start out in a positive light. I had two appointments scheduled—one at 8:40 a.m. for labs followed by a meeting with Dr. Anderson. Then I'd go to my first appointment with the radiation oncologist.

As I was getting ready for these meetings at home, I reflected back to some of the early messages I'd gotten from friends both in writing and in person—"Camille, you're so brave" and "Your courage is amazing." I never really understood why people were saying that, because I didn't feel very brave. I was just doing what I had to do to get rid of this disease, no courage required. Today, I began to understand their comments, because it took a lot of courage to go into the clinic. Knowing that I'd be in appointments until after lunchtime was hard to face. I couldn't bring myself to put on a wig, so I left the house with a bare head.

Once I got to the clinic, instead of stressing in the waiting room, I let my imagination take me away. I pretended I wasn't in a clinic waiting room, but rather an airport, waiting for a flight that would take me away to a warm-weather spa vacation, where I'd meet a group of my favorite girlfriends. As I looked out the window at the gray sky, I smiled because soon I'd be in the warm sun with days of relaxation ahead of me. While it may seem silly, or even slightly insane, it did make me feel better.

Once in the exam room, when Dr. Anderson walked in, he greeted me cheerfully, proclaiming, "You're a TAC survivor!" TAC stands for Taxotere, Adriamycin, and Cytoxan, the three most powerful chemo drugs on the market. Then he gave me some fantastic news: no blood draws during radiation! Then more good news: my port can be removed! The procedure is scheduled for next week! Hurray! He also announced that I'm no longer anemic, but I'll have to keep taking the iron pills until after radiation ends. He gave me one more bit of good news: I don't have to see him until a full week after radiation. So I'll get a weeklong vacation from doctors' appointments after the last radiation treatment. Yippee!

When I went to schedule that post-radiation appointment, plus an appointment for a bone scan, the scheduler removed the round purple "port" sticker from my file. That sight made me smile—I'll be glad when it's out. The bone scan is to get a baseline so they can monitor my bone density over the next few years once hormone therapy begins. In two months, Dr. Anderson and I will make some decisions about what to do—continue to nuke any existing cancer at the expense of my bones, or keep my bones healthy with the risk of leaving any unseen cancer untreated. But I don't need to worry about that now.

After saying good-bye to my oncologist and nurse for the next seven weeks, I went downstairs to radiation to meet with my new best friends. Compared to chemo, I wasn't worried at all about radiation, but after meeting with the radiation oncologist, I'm nervous. I'll go in five days per week for six weeks. Each appointment is about ten minutes, plus another ten to fifteen minutes of waiting, getting into the gown, and getting dressed again. The actual radiation (X rays aimed at my breast) only lasts about two minutes. They don't know why fatigue is a side effect, but the theory is that the body is taxed by just trying to heal from the damage being done each day. The fatigue can start anytime after treatment begins. The treatment itself is painless, but after about three weeks, the skin will burn. I wasn't too worried about burns, because I thought the beams would only be aimed at the spot where my tumor was removed. But today, I learned it's my entire breast, all the way up to above my clavicle. That freaks me out, because it's a much larger area that can be burned.

I also learned some of the possible, but rare, long-term side effects. Because they'll be radiating part of my ribs and a small section of lung, my ribs could be weakened and more prone to breaking, and I could develop some lung conditions. The fact that my bones and lungs are healthy going into radiation means it's unlikely that I'll have these side effects, but it's still scary to hear about the terrible things that can happen.

After scheduling my CT scan, which will help the radiation oncologist determine exactly where the beams should be aimed, I left feeling like rejoicing that chemo is finally over, and I'm onto the next phase of treatment—putting me one step closer to the end of treatment.

The day ended with beautiful snow falling on my bare head. It made everything look clean and white. What started as a scary day ended with beauty and hope.

Four Tattoo Tuesday

Tuesday, March 4, 2008, 8:03 a.m.

Yesterday, I got my first tattoo. Actually, I got four of them. I'm pretty disappointed. They aren't quite as exciting as I expected. Now, it's not what you're probably thinking—I didn't go to a shady tattoo parlor to emerge with an anchor, heart, cross, and dolphin emblazoned on my arm. My tattoos were done at the radiation oncology clinic. They're each the size of the small needle point the technician used to push in the black ink. You'd never know they were there without really looking for them. The tattoos will last forever, and they'll help the radiologist position me on the table each time I go in for treatment.

I also went to yoga yesterday—this is after going to the gym three days in a row. I'm feeling pretty good about getting more exercise. Plenty of exercise will become increasingly important as the ability to manage stress becomes key for doing well at work and being patient with the kids.

I'm stressed now because this afternoon is the port-removal surgery. It's exciting to anticipate having the port out, but I'm nervous for the procedure. Actually, it's not so much the procedure that makes me nervous; it's just that in addition to having my tattoos, which included a CT scan, I also had a DXA bone scan yesterday. Factoring in the port-removal surgery, that will be three appointments in forty-eight hours. It's much like the early days of the diagnosis, when it was one appointment after another. Maybe I'm experiencing a little post-traumatic stress with all these appointments.

When the port is removed, they'll have to start an IV to give me the cocktail for the surgery. It won't quite knock me out, but it will ensure I don't remember what happens in the operating room. This will be the first IV I've had since September. I hate needles. Note: if you hate needles, don't get cancer. So many needles.

Anyway, the best part of my day will be going to work, and I need to leave the house soon. Is that a bad thing or a good thing when the best part of the day is work?

Radiation Details
Wednesday, March 5, 2008, 7:46 p.m.

I thought I'd share more details about the new experiences of my radiology appointment on Monday. The table was very hard; the technician explained that they can't use a padded table, because padding would make it difficult to position me each time. After I lay down on the table, the tech bound my feet together with a huge rubber band. She marked my chest with a black Sharpie. Then the radiation oncologist came in and marked me with a red Sharpie. He added some stickers with wires to my breast. At least it's better than wires *in* my breast, which was the deal in the hours before the lumpectomy. Then the technician gave me the tattoos. The final part was going into the CT scan. Unlike an MRI tube, a CT machine is more like a doughnut. It's noisy—sounds like a plane taking off. The whole experience felt like an alien abduction.

After I left the appointment, I called Wade, who said I sounded depressed. I guess I did feel a little bit depressed. Part of the problem was reading about radiation. While the side effects are nothing like chemo, some radiation effects are lasting. For example, I'll need to be careful to wear sunscreen on the radiated area for the rest of my life; I'll be at risk for skin cancer on the radiated area for the rest of my life. Follow-up care by a radiation oncologist will be necessary for the rest of my life. It's pretty depressing to stare at all those for-the-rest-of-your-life statements.

Lately, I'm feeling angry. Most thirty-eight-year-olds don't have to deal with dozens and dozens of doctors' appointments. I did nothing to deserve this—no smoking, no drinking, no caffeine, no red meat. Anger is one of the stages of grief, and I'm there. It's part of the process, but it feels yucky.

Wade just gave me a wet willy. Jerk. Oh well, I suppose it's a good reality check and a good place to close out this postcard to you all, my home during this difficult Camp Chemo experience.

Cold Snaps and Chemo
Saturday, March 8, 2008, 3:54 p.m.

Girls Scout cookies and muddy paw prints on the kitchen floor are certain signs of spring. Last weekend, both provided hope. The kids were happy to eat the cookies, and our dog, Savannah, was happy to be able to provide her mucky sign of spring. This weekend, we're back to single-digit mornings and below-zero wind chills. Cold snaps and chemo are excellent ways to build character.

Yesterday at the gym, I saw a poster advertising the gym's corporate fitness program. It urged companies to sign up for a wellness plan because it will reduce the company's medical costs. Baloney. I see similar posters at work from our health insurance company. They make me mad. I just don't buy it anymore. I don't eat red meat, don't smoke, don't drink alcohol or caffeine. I go to the gym and eat my veggies. Yet still I got cancer. So whatever.

That being said, I'll continue going to the gym only because it makes me sleep better and helps me manage my emotions. Also, I feel good after a workout. But I won't go to be healthier; I know now we can't control our health even with careful attention to it. Not too long ago, my main objective with exercise was to be healthier; vanity wasn't an issue. Now the objective is to feel good and look better. I'm sick of not looking good. Since my last chemo, I've gained a few pounds. Even my fat clothes aren't fitting comfortably. If I had the cash to buy the next size up, it wouldn't be an issue, but no dice, so I need to trim down.

One thing that's felt really great lately is purging junk from my life. My chemo outfit and all my PJs, which remind me of chemo, have been donated. I've been sorting through boxes of baby things we don't need anymore and donating them, as well. It feels good to make room in my physical space for whatever new is around the corner.

Radiation Tomorrow
Sunday, March 9, 2008, 10:05 p.m.

Radiation starts tomorrow. Five days a week for six weeks. My appointments will be at 7:45 each morning, with an appointment with the radiation oncologist every Wednesday. Each appointment will last about twenty minutes, including waiting room time. The actual radiation will last two minutes. I'm not dreading it the way I dreaded chemo, but it feels like each time I go to a doctor, a little bit of life gets sucked out of me.

I'm worried about possible burns. They're like microwave burns—they burn the tissue from the inside out. The recommendation is to wear a sports bra and be extra gentle with my skin. OK—just another few weeks of trying to figure out what to wear to work with a sports bra. The good news is that I'll finish radiation before Jackson's second birthday.

Going to the gym more regularly has lifted my spirits. I may be feeling ambivalent about the whole idea that a healthy lifestyle makes a difference in disease prevention, but I do feel better when I can at least button my jeans. So to the gym I go.

It's impractical to wear a wig at the gym, so I go with a bandana or nothing on my head. The men seem to look right past me, as if I'm invisible. I seem to strike fear in the eyes of the women. It's a strange feeling to be feared.

At church this morning, all the readings centered on resurrection. Ezekiel saw the dry bones, Jesus raised Lazarus from the dead, and the book of Romans reminded us that "to set the mind on the flesh is death, but to set the mind on the Spirit is life and peace." This resonates with me because as I rebuild my relationship with my body, I remember that despite all my body has been through, my spirit is intact.

Gifts continue to arrive—kind words and prayers and many grocery gift cards. Last week, my yoga teacher gave me a CD of meditations and music she created. It's amazing that people are so generous. Please keep us in your prayers during the final stage of treatment.

Blonde Fun
Tuesday, March 11, 2008, 9:22 p.m.

Do blondes really have more fun? As a lifelong brunette growing up in Minnesota, a.k.a. Little Scandinavia, I've wished for blonde hair. When my search for the perfect wig began, I tried on blonde and red wigs, but neither looked good. It was fall, so my tan was pretty dark. Recently, I attended an American Cancer Society Look Good, Feel Better class and tried a platinum-blonde wig. It looks great! Even Wade likes it. Maybe because my skin is so much lighter from the long winter. Somehow it works. Having almost no eyebrows also helps the blonde make sense. I haven't worn my new wig in public yet, but maybe sometime this weekend? While I wouldn't wear it to a client meeting, it would be fun to wear at work, just to shake things up.

A fellow survivor told me that the Look Good, Feel Better class was a "walk, don't run to it" kind of event. I'm glad I took her advice, and I'm also glad I waited until this point in my treatment to go because I really needed a pick-me-up. Lately, I haven't been feeling great about my appearance, and it made a big difference to play with makeup in a group of fun fellow survivors.

My radiation treatments started yesterday. The treatment itself was fine. I'd been feeling pretty sorry for myself for the past week or two. Yesterday morning, I was feeling much the same way during my treatment. Afterward, I walked back into the waiting room. There, in the waiting room, was a lovely three-year-old girl with no hair, beautiful, big blue eyes, and a Disney-character surgical mask covering her mouth and nose. I went over to say hello. She was whimpering and whining quietly. Her mom said the girl's name is Emma, and she's three. I asked the mom her name too, so I could keep them both in my prayers. As I gently patted her shoulder, she instinctively put her hand up to meet mine. That gesture made it clear to me that many people must be giving her gentle pats lately. After I was safely in my car, I promptly started crying. This beautiful little girl and her sweet mother were going through an awful ordeal. I felt so selfish to be focusing on my own troubles just minutes before meeting Emma and her mom. The day after my diagnosis, I said to Wade, "Thank God it's me and not one of the kids." No parent should have to see their child suffer. Today, during my radiation treatment, I prayed for Emma and her mom.

Meredith

Thursday, March 13, 2008, 11:51 p.m.

Tonight was the public premiere of my new blonde wig! The name she came with is Meredith, but it doesn't do her justice. She's a cross between a modern bob and a pixie. Meredith is cute, smart, and perky enough to work full-time as a television newscaster.

Wade likes the look, Jackson doesn't care, but Vivian is my worst critic. And I quote: "You are not my mommy! You freak! You are not my mommy!" Not quite the reaction I was seeking. Somehow I'll sell her on it . . .

Radiation keeps ticking along. Yesterday as I left the clinic, I was handed a bunch of daffodils courtesy of the American Cancer Society—part of their Daffodil Days fund-raiser. Today, as I left the clinic, I saw little Emma coming in for her treatment. Her dad was with her this time. I asked how she was doing. He said she'd just had a scan, and the news wasn't good. I was afraid to ask what that meant. I told him that they've been in my prayers, and he thanked me. They will, of course, remain in my prayers.

Crud du Jour
Sunday, March 16, 2008, 4:23 p.m.

Week one of radiation is over and no side effects yet. Although cancer hasn't made me sick this week, some big, wet, sloppy kisses from Jackson made all of us sick.

Wednesday night, Jackson was up most of the night with the stomach flu. He was much better by Thursday afternoon. Then Friday night, I was up with the stomach flu. Saturday night, it was Vivian's turn. Nearly two dozen barf sessions between the three of us—many involving clothing, the floor, or bedding. Yuck. Wade hasn't been hungry today, so I'm worried he'll come down with it too. Now Jackson has been barfing all over the house again today. I've been bleaching the house like a crazed housewife on a TV commercial, so hopefully we'll break the puke chain soon.

Vivian cried when we said she couldn't go to church for Palm Sunday today, because she wanted to sing in the children's choir. This was a surprise to me, because normally she fusses about having to go choir practice. Wade did take her to the Children's Theater when she was able to keep her breakfast and lunch down. I stayed home with poor, sick little Jackson. He finally fell asleep for his nap about two hours later than usual.

This weekend, we're a pretty average Minnesota family battling the crud du jour. Not bad to be average for once.

No Bald Photos
Tuesday, March 18, 2008, 10:31 p.m.

This morning, a beautiful snowfall covered everything. The tree branches looked so graceful with the fresh snow. While driving to work, I saw two people building a snowman as they waited for the bus. The best part of a March snowfall in Minnesota is that you know it will soon melt, and today it did melt in the afternoon.

My hair is growing quickly. This should be a 100 percent exciting development, but it gives me pause for one reason. We don't have a photo of me totally bald. The one we have shows me with some stubble, right after Wade shaved my head. If I'm going to have a bald photo, it had better happen soon. The hair I have now isn't enough to show up on a photo. When I first had a shiny bald head, I wanted a photo, but the holidays were upon us, and it just didn't happen. But now my eyebrows are thin, and my eyelashes are skimpy, so getting my picture taken just isn't my idea of a good time. Maybe it's even a good thing that I don't have a photo, because I'm not sure what a photo would accomplish. Strange that I'm so hung up on whether or not there should be a bald photo.

The hair that is starting to grow is in patches of pure white and black. Some areas still have no hair at all—think male-pattern baldness. The hair is very soft and gives me a baby chick appearance, just in time for Easter.

Grown Up Now
Wednesday, March 19, 2008, 9:17 p.m.

On my way home from work today, Wade asked me to stop at the grocery store for hamburgers—one of the few things Vivian will actually eat these days. Very normal seven-year-old behavior. As I rounded the corner to the frozen section, I saw my darling breast surgeon, Dr. Farah, wearing his blue scrubs. I was overjoyed. When I greeted him, I remembered that I was wearing Meredith, so I said my name and reminded him that he'd done my lumpectomy in September when I was a brunette. Not only did he recognize me despite the blonde wig, he apologized for not being able to make it to our art sale on the day of the snowstorm.

Is it typical for patients to love their doctors so much? Before my surgery, I remember remarking that Dr. Farah seemed wonderful, and that's important because you sure don't want some jerk cutting you open. The relationship between a patient and surgeon is special. It's very intimate. Not only has he seen me naked, but he's looked inside me and seen parts of my body I'll never even see. Not to mention that he saved my life. He gets even more bonus points for recommending my beloved oncologist, Dr. Anderson.

Reflecting on seeing Dr. Farah, I realized that when I greeted him in the grocery store today, I was a grown-up, but the first day I met him, just three days after my diagnosis, I was only a child.

Red Aversion

Saturday, March 22, 2008, 9:26 p.m.

My grandmother had a strong aversion to the color blue. We could never give her anything blue for her birthday or Christmas. Even when looking for greeting cards, we'd avoid blue envelopes. We also had to avoid cards that said "To a Special Grandmother" because she thought "special" sounded like the grandmother in the greeting card was mentally challenged. Her reason for despising the color blue wasn't as funny.

One day when my mother was a baby, she stopped breathing and turned blue. My grandmother was panicked, of course. My grandfather ran to the home of a neighbor, who was a doctor. The man revived my mother, her color returned, but my grandmother never forgot that day or the horror of seeing her blue baby.

My own aversion to the color red, which started with the red chemo Adriamycin, isn't as strong as it was a few months ago, but I've decided I'm allowed to avoid that color. The aversion is primarily focused on red liquids, which particularly remind me of the bright-red Adriamycin dripping directly into my veins. Each time after that chemo, I'd pee bright red for a few days as the medicine worked its way through my system. Sometimes my cheeks would turn bright red. Even wearing the color red is something I can't picture doing for quite some time, if ever. Growing up, I couldn't understand why Grandma hated the color blue—until I was old enough to hear the story. Now I can understand, on a more visceral level, her aversion to all things blue. I'm not upset when others wear red; I just don't want that color anywhere on my body. I even threw away all my red nail polish, which used to be a favorite manicure color.

In other news, my car has been acting up. Only thirty-seven thousand miles and the check engine light stayed on all week. On Friday, I brought it into the dealer. With the extended warranty, it's just $100 for them to look at the car and fix it. Vivian and Jackson made the trip with me. While we were waiting for the loaner car, Vivian asked if the complimentary pop in the refrigerated soda case was free. I told her, "No, it's not free. In fact, we're paying $100 just to stand here and look at this pop." Another customer walking by got a good laugh out of that. The dealer loaned me a beautiful, black sports car with leather interior, sunroof, and only twelve hundred miles on it. When they called yesterday to say my car is done, I somehow forgot to call them back. It might be a while before I remember to return the brand-new sporty black car for my tan station wagon with stained seats.

Today, I wore Meredith and, while driving the sports car, I thought how funny to be a blonde driving a sporty black car, when just a few days ago I was a brunette driving a tan station wagon. Things can sure change quickly.

My real hair is growing more each day. Today, as I put lotion on my legs after the shower, I noticed hair on my legs! I hadn't noticed it before because it's so fine, not like the stubble that appears after shaving. Too bad the leg hair didn't just stop growing forever.

Tomorrow, we'll have a small Easter dinner with a few friends and family. Vivian is so excited for Easter. On the day she was born, I looked at her and thought that I'd gladly die to save her. That night, the first night of her life, I dreamed it was Easter morning. In my dream, Vivian was a preschool-aged child, and she was jumping around ecstatic that the Easter Bunny had brought her candy and presents. I'd had several dreams in pregnancy that revealed my fears of becoming a parent (forgetting the baby at the shopping mall, not knowing how to buckle the baby into the car seat), so that dream of Easter morning reassured me; we'd be good parents, capable of making our daughter happy. I wonder if I dreamed about Easter because I'd been thinking I would die for Vivian.

A Quarter Inch of Hair

Saturday, March 29, 2008, 8:07 a.m.

This week marked six months since I had surgery. As life starts to get back to "normal," I realize I'm much more in touch with my mortality. While Dr. Anderson says we're going for a cure, I'm aware there may come a time when I'm given a limit to the number of days I have left to live on earth. So I'm still saving for retirement, but I also know that I'd best not put off things that I'd like to do today. It's sad, but practical. After all, nobody really knows how much time they have to live. After seeing the outpouring of support during the worst of my illness, I have no doubt that my kids would be well cared for, no matter what. And Vivian has proved herself capable of coping with life's most difficult issues.

On a lighter note, Wade and I attended the Minnesota Wild hockey game the other night, and we somehow made it onto TV in a crowd shot with me as a blonde!

At this point, I have about a quarter inch of hair, which doesn't amount to much. Considering that hair generally grows about a half inch per month, it could be early summer before I can do anything with it. For some reason, I thought that once it started growing back, I could ditch the wigs immediately. I'm going to have to wait just a while longer, though.

My eyebrows are starting to grow back. Today, for the first time in six months, I plucked a few stray eyebrow hairs. Yikes! I'd forgotten how much that hurts! My eyes were watering up, and I could only do four or five before I had to stop. I've yet to take a razor to my legs because it's still too cold for shorts or skirts. I wonder if I'll cut myself shaving like when I was a teen first learning to shave my legs.

I've been feeling great about getting back to the gym on a more regular basis. When the surgeon told me I shouldn't lift weights because my lymph nodes were removed, I was worried. But now I think, why not? I've been lifting weights since I was fifteen. My dad, who died from a smoking-related cancer when I was young, was a bodybuilder, so it's in my blood. I can't live life without lifting weights. I don't care what the surgeon told me. The weight I'm lifting is half of what I was able to do prediagnosis. But it's a start.

Understatement
Monday, March 31, 2008, 6:36 p.m.

Yesterday, Vivian and I went swimming at an indoor pool. Now I'm listening to Vivian and two of her friends sing songs from *High School Musical* as they play with Legos. It's lovely to spend time together, but it does make me a little blue to realize all I missed when I was recovering from the lumpectomy and chemo.

A few nights ago, I had a strange dream. I ran into someone I haven't seen since my diagnosis. I walked up to him and said, "I have cancer." It made me realize that somehow I've never said those words out loud. I tell people, "I had a lumpectomy" or "I had chemo for breast cancer." Early on, I decided to use language that put the cancer in the past tense. But this dream made me realize how dramatic it is to say, "I have cancer."

Maybe it's connected to the Minnesotan reliance on understatement. Even my doctor didn't say, "You have cancer." Instead, he called and said, "You have lobular carcinoma, which can be cancer or precancer." A little later in the conversation, I asked him when we'd know if it's cancer or precancer. "It's cancer," he admitted. Perhaps because he never directly stated it as "You have cancer," I was calmer about the whole thing. Possibly his abstract language help me bypass some of the fear.

Failing the (Genetic) Test
Thursday, April 3, 2008, 7:39 p.m.

Yesterday, the genetic counselor called to say she should have results from the BRCA1 and BRCA2 (breast cancer genetic mutation) test today. When I had the blood draw for the test, I was hoping I'd test positive for the mutation so at least I could know the cause of my cancer. But in the last few days, I've been hoping I don't have the mutation because it would lead to difficult decisions about my future care, and I don't want the kids to inherit the mutation.

Well, the genetic counselor called today, and as it turns out, yes, I have the BRCA2 genetic mutation. What does this mean? I don't know. She starting telling me various statistics on the phone, but my head was spinning. I actually felt dizzy as I walked away from my desk to call Wade.

Wade and I are meeting with the genetic counselor tomorrow to get more perspective. We'll also talk with Dr. Anderson in a few weeks, and I'm sure he'll have some recommendations. The genetic counselor told me on the phone that this explains why I got the cancer—that it's not my fault. She also said it means that my risk of ovarian cancer is higher than normal. While I don't need to get my ovaries removed in the next twenty minutes, the counselor said she'd be upset if at age forty-eight I still have them. I'm not sure if BRCA2 is the one that means I may need to consider mastectomy. I just can't think about that right now. We'll get more information tomorrow and take it from there.

The genetic counselor also said she can help me draft a letter to my family explaining about BRCA2 and what it could mean to them. It makes me think about when someone gets a venereal disease and they have to call everyone they've ever slept with to tell them the news. Now I have to send a VD letter to my whole family. We don't know if the genetic mutation is from my mother's or father's side. If anyone wants to get tested, the letter will advise of the various options. If you're one of the few blood relatives of mine who reads this, consider yourself notified. You'll get a VD letter in the mail soon. Sorry about that.

Just last night, I was telling Wade that I'm glad all of this is almost behind us and that I still feel like a pretty healthy person. Now I find out I'm a genetic mutant.

Jackson is throwing his gigantic rubber ball from the Easter Bunny at me right now, so I guess it's time for the mutant to play.

Mutant Dreams
Friday, April 4, 2008, 7:31 a.m.

Last night, I dreamed my car was vandalized three times. The third time it was winter, and the entire roof disappeared from the car, making it vulnerable to cold and snow. Wade and I were trying to figure out who did it. We were finding clues but could never figure it out.

Another transparent dream. The car represents my body (the vehicle in which humans travel through life) and the vandalism is pretty self-explanatory. Finding clues about who did this to me is the genetic testing, but we couldn't pin the deed on one side of the family just yet.

While Wade and I were searching for clues in the dream, we walked past several parents, each with a child. In each case, the parent was giving the child a gift that turned out to be a card with money. Not the exciting gift the child wanted to receive. Someday I'll have to get my kids tested for the BRCA2 gene, which I now know they have a 50 percent chance of carrying. Not the kind of inheritance I wanted to give my kids.

The night wasn't all weird dreams. The Minnesota Wild won and clinched the division title. It was a great game. Good thing they're going to the playoffs; I need something to look forward to in the next few weeks.

Mutant Status
Sunday, April 6, 2008, 10:00 p.m.

After talking with the genetic counselor, I'm way less freaked out about the whole mutant thing. She explained in detail what the findings mean. The bottom line is that I'll need to have my ovaries removed due to my increased risk of ovarian cancer. This won't be a big deal because the surgery is laparoscopic, meaning the incisions are tiny and the recovery time is just a few days. She gave me the name of a good oncology gynecological surgeon. She also explained that I should make sure they know I have the BRCA2 mutation—they'll do the pathology differently with that knowledge.

My mother has agreed to have the BRCA2 genetic test. She wasn't at all freaked out by hearing I have the mutation. As a retired registered nurse, she thinks this is all so fascinating from a medical perspective. My mom has sympathy for me, of course, but I'm glad she's able to look at this issue as a health care professional, rather than as a layperson who might be really disturbed by this information. Within a few months of the test, we should know if I inherited the gene from my mom or my dad. Then my cousins on the offending side can decide if they'd like to have the test, as well.

The other big decision I'll need to make is what to do about my breasts. (That sounds really weird, doesn't it?!) The genetic counselor explained that my risk for getting a new breast cancer goes up by 2 percent each year. My risk was going up only 1 percent per year before the test. I think it tops out at an 85 percent chance of getting a new breast cancer. About one-third of all women who test for the BRCA2 mutation but don't have cancer yet opt for prophylactic mastectomy. It's considered prophylactic because they haven't experienced cancer yet, so the mastectomy is preventative. About half of women who have the BRCA2 mutation and have cancer will have the mastectomy. So I'm in the fifty-fifty group. At this point, having the ovaries removed seems like a no-brainer. Ovarian cancer is asymptomatic until it's quite advanced, and the screening isn't reliable. We're done having children, so I don't feel so sad having them removed. Plus, I'll have to remove the ovaries chemically or have them surgically destroyed to stop the estrogen, anyway, because my cancer is estrogen receptive, which means estrogen is its main source of energy. So surgery to remove the ovaries seems like the best option. But thinking about a mastectomy is another matter. It's major surgery with a long recovery time. If I go that route, though, I'd want reconstruction, which is another three or four painful procedures. I can't even imagine that much surgery anytime soon.

Maybe someday mastectomy will be a viable option for me, but right now I trust the current screening for breast cancer (mammogram, followed by an MRI in six months, repeat forever). I've already found a lump once, the one that led to my diagnosis, so I trust that I'd find another if it shows up.

Wade and I went out on Friday night. On Saturday, Vivian had a dance performance. Today, she attended the first meeting of her book group for little girls. The girls all read *Black Beauty* and had quite a good discussion. I was impressed. They'll read *Little House in the Big Woods* next. Vivian began bugging me for her own book group at age five, so I'm glad I finally created one for her. After a week of being immersed in my new mutant status, this weekend seemed so normal.

Radiation Burns
Tuesday, April 8, 2008, 9:03 p.m.

Only one and a half weeks left of radiation. That's good, because I'm starting to feel sleepy early in the evening now. I'm also starting to get burned. I have one purple patch of burned skin under my right arm. My entire right breast is red, and the pores are nearly black. The tissue feels more firm than usual. It hurts to lie on my right side. It occurs to me that after radiation ends, I'll still have the burns, and I wonder how long it will take for them to heal.

Soon after my lumpectomy, I experienced a lymphedema symptom called cording. As the name suggests, one of the lymphatic vessels becomes tight and appears tough, like a cord beneath the skin. It's as painful and disconcerting as it sounds. Now, the cording in my right arm has returned. I've been doing the massage on my arm the physical therapist at showed me, but it isn't working, so I need to go back there to have a professional work it out.

Driving to radiation every morning at 7:45 is getting old. I've been going every day for four and a half weeks already. Because I'm so fatigued, I've moved my radiation appointments to afternoons for the rest of this week. I'll be able to sleep in a little bit for the next few mornings. Next week is going to be pretty busy at work, so I'll have to keep my morning appointments and just get to bed earlier.

Yesterday, we went as a family to the first of a four-week series of Facing Cancer Together (FACT), a service of the Angel Foundation of

Minnesota. We did yoga as a family and then ate dinner with the other families. After dinner, the kids went with volunteers to do crafts and discuss how cancer has changed their families. The adults went to a support group. We really only had time to tell our stories, but for a few minutes, we discussed how to best communicate our various cancer situations with our children.

Wade found it pretty depressing to hear some of these stories. It's a lot to process all at once. One woman was in a wheelchair because her breast cancer metastasized to her spine, brain, and bone marrow. Another had ordered a wheelchair but found her walking later improved. A few people with pancreatic cancer had been told they have limited time left. Some others have long outlived their original prognosis. A few of us are on our first time with cancer, while the majority have metastatic cancers. Everyone in the group is fighting the disease with great faith and hope. I'm inspired.

Last week, I visited the dentist. It had been six months, so they didn't know about my diagnosis. It was weird to tell people who don't already know the whole cancer story. The dentist asked if I'd been experiencing dry mouth. My mouth hasn't felt dry, but my breath has seemed bad to me the last few weeks. Based on that and what he observed during the exam, he said I do have dry mouth, and he gave me some mouthwash and toothpaste that should help.

Dry mouth is something that would have really bugged me a year ago, but now it's something I've adjusted to with little notice. Dry mouth is such a small thing compared to the severe fatigue and many other symptoms I've experienced.

Radiation Bonus Week

Wednesday, April 9, 2008, 6:48 p.m.

My weekly appointment with the radiation oncologist was today. I mentioned something about being done with radiation a week from Friday, to which he replied, "No." He said that it's really seven weeks that I'm doing, not six weeks. I flashed back to the day of my lumpectomy—lying on the table, having wires stuck into my tumor before the surgery. After the doctor put one wire in, he explained there was a miscommunication between him and the surgeon: I actually had two tumors instead of just one! At that time, I was hours away from being numbed up, so I was in no position to complain about it. I wouldn't have prepared any differently for the surgery had I known it was two tumors instead of one, anyway.

An extra week of radiation, which I'm trying to think of as a bonus week, means another week without wearing necklaces (I just have to remove them for radiation, anyway), another week of going to the clinic every single day to disrobe, and another week of a disgusting metal taste in my mouth during the treatment. When I asked why I had to go for seven weeks, he gave me this disturbing answer: "Your margins were close, and you're really young." The being young I can understand, since he means that presumably I have more years to live, thus more time for reoccurrence. The part about "close margins" is disturbing because I've never heard that before. After the lumpectomy, I thought they'd said the margins were good.

When my surgeon explained what would happen during my lumpectomy, he told me that they would do pathology on the tumor to make sure they got a centimeter margin of healthy tissue around the entire tumor. If they couldn't accomplish that the first time around, it could mean I'd have to go back a few days later for a mastectomy. Luckily, after the pathology report came back, the surgeon came into my hospital room and announced that he got the margins. So I assumed everything was cool. Now to hear "close margins" from the radiation oncologist—I'm not sure what to think. I'll see Dr. Farah after I'm done with radiation. He should be able to provide some answers.

Today, the nurse gave me a cream for the burns and said I can use cold compresses on them. She also suggested taking ibuprofen for pain and inflammation. She said I should listen to my body and rest when I need to rest. While this is true, I also explained that I feel really good being at work because it fuels me. In the next few weeks, I'll have to find that balance again between resting my body and feeding my soul.

Some of these setbacks—like the discovery of the BRCA2 mutation and now an extra week of radiation—are getting to me a little bit. I'm not really upset so much as exhausted. I'm so ready to have my energy back. Wah, wah, wah, poor me. Overall, I have more to be happy about than to complain about, but still. Hopefully, one day, communication between doctor and patient will leave no surprises.

Science-Fiction Radiation

Tuesday, April 15, 2008, 8:45 p.m.

Dr. Anderson called the other day to ask, "Why didn't you call me once you got the genetic test results?" I thought to myself, *Why would I call you?!* and *How do you know I got the results?!* Turns out, he was anxious to discuss my ovaries, tubes, and uterus. What a guy. He recommends all three be removed. He suggested two surgeons to "interview" and see which I prefer. He also cleared me to have the ovaries, tubes, and uterus surgery as soon as my radiation is done. While we talked, I cracked some jokes and made him laugh. As he caught his breath, he said, "You're like a sister to me!" Now that's a good position to be in with your doctor! As for the surgery, my plan is to do it as quickly as possible.

The bad news from Dr. Anderson is that a different genetic test he ordered—to help inform our decisions on which drugs are likely to be most effective moving forward—came back without a clear answer. We'll have to weigh the pros (deleting all estrogen from my system, giving any remaining cancer no fuel) and cons (risking osteoporosis from a lack of estrogen) of the most likely course of treatment.

With hindsight, I can say I sailed through the first four weeks of radiation. Week five was another story. My pain level has been increasing. Under my arm is the worst part. This is quite common, because friction under the arm is inevitable and problematic for radiated skin. I've been taking a couple of ibuprofen per day, which has helped. But sleeping at night is difficult. Imagine a really bad sunburn. My skin is red like that, but also each hair follicle is black. Some of my skin has started peeling.

Beneath the visible burns, the tissue is sore because it's burned too. It hurts more and more when I try to lift my right arm above my head. At the gym, any exercise that engages the chest muscle has been deleted from my workout. I thought I might have to have to quit my workouts altogether because I've been so drained. All weekend, I went to bed early and took naps but still felt tired.

Yesterday, I whined to my radiation oncologist, and he said he could write a note if I don't feel I can work full-time. I pooh-poohed that idea, but I do worry I'll have to start going home early. Then the nurse put a pain medication patch under my arm and—voilà!—the pain was magically gone! I slept great last night.

I went to the integrative health center at the hospital today and bought some oils that a fellow survivor insisted would help with the radiation burns. Just one application of the oils and my skin already looks better! As a bonus, the key essential oils—helichrysum, frankincense, lavender, and geranium—smell beautiful.

Here's a glimpse into the sci-fi world of radiation. Everything starts out like a normal doctor visit. The waiting-room television is blaring either *Good Morning America* or *The View*, no matter what time of day I'm there. Most everyone in the waiting room is older than I am. Soon after arriving, I'm called by one of the six radiation technicians. They're on a rotation, so I never know whose head will pop out of the door and say my name. We chitchat as we walk back to the cavernous treatment room. I undress from the waist up behind a curtain that doesn't fully pull shut. At my first few treatments, I'd use one of the gowns, but I soon opted for a towel instead. There's no point putting on a gown. It comes right off on the table, anyway. Plus, the towel provides more warmth.

I lie down on a bed of Plexiglas with a towel over it. At least two radiation therapists stay with me. Sometimes a resident attends, as well. My pillow is just a plastic form to keep my head in place. My Plexiglas bed moves up on a hydraulic lift as if I'm a Chevy in need of tire rotation. A bolster is slid under my knees, and one of the therapists puts a large rubber band around my feet to immobilize them. I immobilize my arms by grabbing a T bar over my head. Picture gels cover three of the huge fluorescent lights on the ceiling. The gels depict a lovely mountain scene. I can't really see it because my head is turned to my left side. I have to peek up at it sideways if I want a little glimpse of what I'm missing in the Alps.

After I'm all immobilized and "comfy" on my Plexiglas bed, the huge x-ray machine begins to move over to my left side until the machine is all I can see. The technicians start adjusting the bed up and down, back and forth while muttering phrases I don't understand like: "I need a two lift," "I need to open my jaws," "Nine point seven. Ninety-seven. Nine point seven. Ninety-seven," and "Move to the super clav."

Meanwhile, they stand over me like space aliens, staring at my chest, finding my sternum and clavicle with their fingers, looking closely for my tiny tattoos to find the perfect position for the radiation. One of the technicians clearly smokes because I can smell it on his skin as he gets close to align me correctly. At one point, someone takes out a small ruler and holds it on my chest to make sure I measure up to the ray of red light coming from the machine. While all this is happening, the thirty-odd fluorescent and incandescent lights in various areas of the room flick on and off. It goes from bright light to perfectly dark to bright again.

Finally, they turn off the lights for good and say, "Here we go." They leave the room for another room down the hall where they can see and hear me on television screens. Their room is lined in lead, so they're safe from the radiation. Then a light on the machine turns on, and a loud buzzing starts. One Mississippi, two Mississippi, three Mississippi, all the way to twelve Mississippi.

Then they come back in to rearrange me while the machine rotates to the left side. This is my favorite position because from this angle I can read the warning stickers on the machine—"Caution" and "Avoid exposure." My favorite. Yes, I wish I could avoid exposure. The techs leave the room again (to avoid exposure), the light goes on, the loud buzz starts and continues for one Mississippi, two Mississippi, three Mississippi up to twelve, thirteen, or twenty. Depends on the day. If I haven't already started to taste it, a yucky metallic taste forms in the very back of my throat.

The technicians come back and rearrange me for the final position. This time, the machine is directly above my chest. Before they leave, they put a piece of tape on my right ribs to pull the skin taut so the radiation doesn't get stuck in a pocket of flesh and ruin the skin even more than it already does. That's why all my hair follicles in the radiated area look like black dots; the radiation bounces around in those pockets and causes more damage than if it just goes over a smooth surface.

As soon as the buzzing stops (somewhere around twelve Mississippi), I remove the tape and pull my legs up to my chest to remove the rubber band holding my feet. That's except for one day of the week when they have to take some X rays too, so I need to stay still. The X rays last for just one Mississippi. I need to wait until they return to the room before I can sit up. The machine is still directly above me, and I'm still up on the lift, so if I do dare sit up, my head will hit the machine. When they enter the room, they move the machine and lower me slowly on the hydraulic lift. I return to the curtain that doesn't completely shut, put on my clothes, and call out, "See you tomorrow."

Today was my final day of this routine. Tomorrow, my "boost" will start. That involves aiming the radiation only at my surgical scar, not the entire breast. The radiation oncologist will be in to help position me properly. This routine will last until a week from Friday. I'm in the home stretch!

Coyote

Monday, April 21, 2008, 7:43 p.m.

People are always telling me about their survivor friend's post-chemo hair growth. Usually it's someone who gets darker, curly hair. So I've been imagining my hair growing back black and curly. Instead, my one-inch hairs are gray and white. I look more like Jamie Lee Curtis than the wild, gorgeous gypsy of my imagination. Even my eyebrows are gray. But beggars can't be choosers.

Last week, I ditched the wig for a day to raise money for Race for the Cure, Team Camille. My coworkers donated more than $200—so now the total raised by Team Camille is over the $1,000 mark. I'm so proud to be raising money to help breast cancer research. It also felt good to go wigless. It's amazing to have enough hair to feel the wind blow through it again.

My right breast is a freak show. The peeling burns reveal paper-thin skin beneath. I've counted six different skin tones on my breast. The magic essential oils are making a big difference in the pain, which only remains under my arm. Walking to my car today, I noticed a scar on the parking lot pavement that revealed layers of older pavement beneath. I decided that it looks like the layers of scars on the skin of my breast.

Last week, Wade's back went out, so I came home to watch Jackson while he was at the chiropractor. It was a beautiful day, so Jackson and I immediately went outside. We walked up the sidewalk enjoying the sunshine. A good deal of time was spent marveling at sticks and pulling petals off flowers. As we stood on the sidewalk, a man walked his dog across the street. Then out of nowhere came another dog, off its leash and running toward us. I always take notice of loose dogs right away because we have a leash law. This dog was pale, with long fur. She resembled a husky. As she paused in the yard two houses up from us, I realized this wasn't a domestic dog. It looked like a wolf, but she was too small. As she bounced out of sight, I yelled to the man walking his dog, "What was that?"

"A coyote," he replied.

"I hope she makes her way to the river," I said, considering the many blocks and busy intersections she'd have to travel to make it.

"She's headed in the right direction," the man said, and we continued on our separate ways.

The beauty of this creature is impossible to describe. She took my breath away. As Jackson and I continued, all at once, illness and injury made a kind of sense to me. Had Wade not needed the chiropractor that morning, I never would have seen that lovely creature. Peace enveloped me as we continued to walk and marvel at the spring plants. So much has been revealed to me in the course of my illness. I've experienced things that never would have happened were it not for the misfortune of one rogue gene. That isn't to say I'm happy about it but rather that an unexpected coyote sighting gave me a dusty glimpse into making meaning of illness and the peace that can take its place.

Learning Experience

Sunday, April 27, 2008, 9:38 p.m.

People keep asking me what I've learned from this whole experience. Here are some things I've learned so far:

Blondes don't have more fun.

Nurses are angels on earth.

Push handicap-accessible door buttons, rather than reaching for door handles. (That's what all the doctors and nurses do in the hospital. They must know something we don't know.)

Doctors deserve every penny they earn.

Worry is worthless.

Prayer works.

There is nothing to fear but fear itself.

I'm about to remove myself from the prayer lists at both my mom's and my own churches, because I feel like I'm in the home stretch.

This weekend, we attended a fund-raiser for Vivian's school. It was taxing to make small talk. I want to be honest and have conversations about real things, not restaurants, vacations, and movies. After attending the school fund-raiser, I'm questioning how much I want to be back in the normal world. I feel myself leaving a world where I could say anything and dip into the realm of real feelings with others. Now I'm moving back to the superficial world, and I'm not so sure I like it . . .

Chess with the Devil
Thursday, May 8, 2008, 8:29 p.m.

Meeting with Dr. Anderson today was much more difficult than I imagined. For some reason, I thought we'd be discussing my poor memory, hot flashes, and so on, but none of that came up. It quickly became a very heavy conversation.

He counseled me about which medication I should take. While there are no clear and obvious choices, we agreed on the aromatase inhibitor, in the form of a daily pill, for five years, and then tamoxifen, also a daily pill, for the rest of my life. These medications will stop any remaining estrogen from flowing. The aromatase inhibitor will lower my bone density, though, and put me at risk for osteoporosis. I'll have a bone scan on Monday so they can start monitoring it annually. My bones got a whooping a few years back when I had thyroid trouble, so I'm going to need to learn what I can do to improve them. I already do weight-bearing exercise, so that should help.

Then we got to the really heavy stuff. We agreed that the ovaries, tubes, and uterus have to go. The reason to remove the ovaries and tubes is to help prevent my primary breast cancer from metastasizing by eliminating the main source of estrogen. Plus, my BRCA2 status makes it a no-brainer, because that status puts me at a higher-than-normal risk for ovarian cancer. Taking out the uterus is advised because another side effect of the aromatase inhibitor is an increased risk of uterine cancer. All these things will also prevent my existing cancer from metastasizing, or invading other organs in my body. As Dr. Anderson said, if that happens, then it's game over. They'd be able to prolong my life, but I would ultimately die of breast cancer.

The big question he needs me to answer is, should I keep my breasts? I have a high percentage chance of getting a new breast cancer. Having a double mastectomy will reduce my chance of getting a new breast cancer by 85 percent. The genetic counselor left me with the impression that as long as I have trust in the MRI and mammogram screenings, I can keep my breasts. However, today I realized that even if the screenings work, they could still reveal a new cancer. While it would be treatable, I'd still have to do surgery, chemo, and radiation all over again. Reducing that chance of a new cancer from 85 percent to just 15 percent is looking pretty attractive.

As I talked to Dr. Anderson, I said, "This all seems so serious."

"This is very serious," he admitted.

Sometimes when the phone rings, I pretend it's Dr. Anderson calling to tell me this has all been a terrible mistake—I never had cancer in the first place. He also informs me that they want to give us a million dollars so we won't sue for malpractice. Sometimes when I'm sitting in the clinic waiting room, I pretend I'm a pharmaceutical sales rep, not a patient. But being face-to-face with Dr. Anderson telling me we have to be aggressive or it's "game over" and removing my breasts will prevent new cancers is a slap of reality. I'm thrown back into the world of statistics where I have to make painful numerical decisions designed to maintain my life. It feels like playing chess with the devil.

When I returned to the waiting room to sit until they called me for my labs, I felt like I'd been sucker-punched and all the wind was knocked out of me. On the other side of the waiting room, a man was reassuring his companion that faith can overcome disease. She'd just been told she'll need chemo again. The man told four stories about him laying hands on someone, praying to Jesus, and the person being healed. Part of me felt resentful that he was trying to convince his companion that all she needs is faith. After all, it takes doctors and science too. He kept saying, "The doctors only know what they learned in college, I put my faith in the God that created me out of dust." The other part of me wanted to go up to him and ask him to lay hands on me so I can be healed once and for all. Instead, I went for my labs.

My natural inclination is to go along with whatever Dr. Anderson suggests. Mind you, he won't say, "You should have a mastectomy." However, the numbers he presents make a compelling case. Wade is a bit more skeptical. We talked about getting a second opinion about the mastectomy. I don't need to make the decision right away, but within the next few years, I'll need to decide.

Next week, I'll meet with a surgeon to discuss the ovaries, tubes, and uterus removal. My main concern is how much time I'll have to take off work. I need to consider the time it will take to heal and the amount of pain management that will be required.

I've also decided to meet with a breast surgeon and a plastic surgeon to discuss mastectomy and reconstruction. That way I'll learn exactly what is involved. I've heard terrible things about reconstruction—it's multiple procedures, it's very painful, it takes a long time. Meeting with surgeons will give me a more specific idea of what to expect.

We aren't going to discuss any of this with Vivian until after we have details on the date of surgery, how many days in the hospital, and how long the recovery will take. The counselor at our Facing Cancer Together support group suggested we not burden Vivian with partial information. Kids need concrete information whenever possible. The last time I went to the hospital, we told her I'd be home by the end of the day. It turned out I stayed in the hospital for three nights, and then I was very sick for several days at home, and then I had one round of chemo after another. This time, we want to prepare her for what's most likely to happen so she doesn't have any more unhappy surprises. Or at least we can minimize them.

My entire family wants to be reassured that I'm going to be OK, but I can't give that reassurance. It's not clear to me I'll be OK.

Worry Machine

Mother's Day, Sunday, May 11, 2008, 9:25 p.m.

The late-night worry machine is back. The past few nights I've been up with a sore throat and stuffy nose. Then I get to thinking, which isn't the right thing to do late at night.

Our support-group counselor often said that when it's obvious something is happening, it's important to tell children what's going on. If you don't, they'll imagine something much worse than the reality. I think I'm being like a child now—filling in the blanks of all these possible surgeries with more scary imaginings than is probably real. However, after having surgery, I know there's pain, and I dread it.

With my lumpectomy, chemo, and radiation, I had this fighting mentality that made everything bearable. When I thought everything was over, I was ready to rest. But all of a sudden, I need to go back into a battle I was never prepared for in the first place. Normally, I'm so positive, but in the middle of the night, it's impossible to be positive. On top of that, my faith is nowhere to be found. I sense that saying a few prayers will bring it back, but for some reason, prayer just isn't an appealing option right now. So strange to feel this way, but that's where I am with my faith. I often recall a quote by Blaise Pascal that says there's a God-shaped hole in everyone's soul. While that hole is feeling pretty empty right now, I'm resisting allowing God back in. It's almost like wanting to refuse my medicine: I know it's good for me, but I just want to pretend I don't need it. This is my late-night life, but the daytime is filled with wonderful distractions. The beauty of the world is revealed in the daylight.

Today was filled with the best distractions. It started with the Race for the Cure with nearly fifty thousand people walking and running. Last year, $2.3 million was raised, and I'm sure the total will be even more this year. I walked in a sea of pink with several coworkers, all very strong women. Having them there to support me was amazing. As we walked, the hope in that crowd was palpable. The survivors' celebration afterward included a tradition of having women stand who have survived after forty years, thirty years, twenty years, ten years, five years, and one year. One little woman was a sixty-two-year survivor. Seeing these old women inspired me. Despite our youth-oriented culture, I long to grow old.

After the race, Vivian and I went to the Children's Theater to see *The Magic Mrs. Piggle Wiggle*. Hearing Vivian laugh out loud had to be the best Mother's Day gift! Then having little Jackson give out kisses freely at dinner with my own mom was also wonderful. The little man is normally quite stingy with his kisses, but I got two yesterday, and my mom got one.

Even as the distraction of the day dissolves into the worry of the night, I know the sun will rise soon, and the happy distractions of waking life will return.

Community

Sunday, May 18, 2008, 6:21 p.m.

Today, I'm thinking about community. I've been reflecting on all different kinds of community and how they've been helping our family cope over the past eight months. Community is more than simple group membership; it's an unwritten contract of agreeing to help one another. I'm so happy to be part of many strong communities.

Community doesn't need to be a formal group; it can be based on proximity like a neighborhood or a workplace. Because we share the same space, it's so important to support one another, and that happens best when we know one another. While on a walk today, I realized that each person I passed shared the same human experiences of intense joy and terrible suffering. The longer I live on borrowed time, the more I realize the only really important things are helping each other and making this journey more enjoyable for those who share our travels.

It all seems so simple today. The sun has been shining for the past five days, we've had a very relaxing weekend, and I had enough money in my pocket to buy Vivian ice cream today.

This brightness is a sharp contrast to the last few weeks that have seemed so intense and dark. While I still have some big decisions to make, I'm realizing that there aren't any decisions that need to be made this minute.

Last week, I met with an oncology gynecological surgeon, Dr. Beckman. She explained how the ovaries, tubes, and uterus would be removed laparoscopically with four tiny incisions measured in millimeters. The decision to have the uterus removed is a coin toss, but there's no reason to keep it, so I'll have it removed too. I'm done with it, and if it can grow cancer, let's ditch it. The procedure will mean at least one night in the hospital. Then I'll need two weeks off work. After two weeks, I can return part-time for one week, and then full-time. Then, it will take another three to four weeks before I feel 100 percent. I liked Dr. Beckman, and I feel ready to choose her as my surgeon.

One option she laid out is that if I plan a mastectomy and reconstruction, all three surgeries can be done at one time. This is a very attractive option to me, because I'd rather serve concurrent recovery sentences than consecutive ones.

On Wednesday, I'll meet which Dr. Farah, my breast surgeon, to discuss the mastectomy and find out which plastic surgeons he recommends.

As Wade and I wrapped up the conversation with Dr. Beckman, she told me to take my time deciding on the mastectomy; there's no hurry. I left her office feeling totally resolved to do the mastectomy and reconstruction. But then by this morning, I didn't feel so sure—showering, wearing my gym clothes, and working out all had me really considering what it would be like to not have my breasts. It's hard for me to know if I'm reconsidering a mastectomy or if I'm just sad about the whole thing.

The difference between uncertainty and mourning feels quite small. Am I really uncertain about having the mastectomy? Or am I simply sad about the loss of a part of my body that has served me well by feeding both of my children?

Unattractive Options

Wednesday, May 21, 2008, 7:48 p.m.

Driving to see Dr. Farah, the breast surgeon, today, I was so nervous I was almost shaking. I even cried in his office. When he asked what was upsetting me (besides the obvious cancer thing), I couldn't articulate it. Some women wish for different breasts. I've never been unhappy with mine. A few years ago, I was at a baby shower, and everyone was bemoaning the fact that after having children their breasts had lost their perkiness. I kept my mouth shut, because mine perked right back after both kids. They've never been too big or too small. If I was a person interested in plastic surgery, breasts would be the last place I'd start. Instead, I'd start with a nose job. Aside from my feelings about my body, I just simply don't want to have a mastectomy. I don't want to keep my breasts, either. I don't want to have reconstruction, but I don't want to "go flat" as Dr. Farah puts it.

If Camp Chemo were a real place, right now it would feel like a prison camp, a place I was forced to go and can't leave. A dreadful place where none of my options are attractive.

Dr. Farah warned me that doing the hysterectomy, oophorectomy, mastectomy, and reconstruction at one time would make for a very long surgery, and the risk of blood clots would increase. He also explained all the places on my body, including chest, belly, and back, that would be sore, and it might be too much pain to properly manage all at once. Even his body language communicated that he thought while it's *possible* to do all the procedures at once, it's not the best idea. When Dr. Beckman had mentioned the option of all the procedures at once, her example was of a mother of an ill child, which was the only reason she chose to do all the surgeries at once. I only want to do them together for my convenience, but if the recovery time and risk of complications increases, I'd rather split up the procedures. Wade really wants me to split them up because he thinks all of them together would be overwhelming.

I know now I'll have the mastectomy, but I feel relieved that I don't have to do it right away. I also feel relieved that I can fast-track removing the ovaries, tubes, and uterus, because I don't have to coordinate it with breast surgery. I'm weirdly anxious to get my ovaries removed. I'm so afraid the pathology report will reveal ovarian cancer.

It was difficult to shake off the appointment with the Dr. Farah and get back to work, but once I got going, I felt the world normalize and my mood improved. Then tonight, as I went for a walk alone with Jackson, who fell asleep in his stroller, the heaviness returned. It's like a black cloud hanging over me, like an actual weight on my shoulders. It's physical. Even chatting with neighbors feels strained, while normally I might converse for hours with anyone who'd tolerate my chattiness. Toward the end of my walk, it hit me: I'm dropping back down into that other plane of existence, the same place I went during chemo. It's that thin place where the border between the physical world and spirit world becomes blurred. It's a place where only the most important things matter. Getting grounded in the details of this world is difficult right now, but at the same time, staying connected to them is perhaps more important than ever. Once again, my salvation will be balance.

My prayer life is still nonexistent. The barrier to God is such a mystery. Maybe on some level, I'm feeling anger, so I have to shut off communication with God. Recently, I've realized that while I have no interest in prayer, others are still (thank heaven) praying for me. I believe that God works through people, and all the kindness around me is an expression of his love. So even though I'm not praying, I'm happy to know others are praying for me.

Mutant Protection
Thursday, May 22, 2008, 10:04 p.m.

The uterus, ovaries, and tubes removal is set for June 3. I was nearly giddy after scheduling the procedure. A huge weight has been lifted. While I don't look forward to the recovery time, I'm excited to have it on the calendar, which means I know when it will be over. I'll also feel so happy when I hear the news my organs are free of cancer. Knock on wood. If they do find cancer during the operation, they'll immediately open me up and dig around for more. After surgery, if the final dissection and pathology finds cancer, I'll need another surgery eight weeks later. Statistically, there's only a 2 percent chance they'll find anything, so I can safely feel confident.

The ovary removal is the last procedure for treating my primary cancer. This will stop most of the estrogen in my body. The medication I'm taking now should stop any remaining estrogen. So if there are any cancer cells hanging out, they'll be starved of the estrogen they need to grow.

Vivian will still be in school for a few days after the surgery, and then with the first few days of summer vacation, I hope she'll be happily distracted while I recover.

Wade's sister who lives in Brooklyn, Carlene, arrived today with her two kids, Konner and Tessa. They drove to Iowa, where Wade and Carlene and their brothers, Kent and Mark, grew up. Vivian, Jackson, and I will join them in Iowa tomorrow night. On Saturday, we'll celebrate our niece Amanda's high school graduation. I'm looking forward to seeing everyone and congratulating Amanda. In the past few months, I've really started having an increased appreciation for these life-cycle events. My cousin Kelsey's wedding shower was so much fun a few weeks ago. Before cancer, I didn't really understand the big deal about wedding showers, graduations, and so on, and sometimes these events would feel like a big disruption. Now I'm thrilled to have reasons to celebrate. I can appreciate that high school graduation and the transition to college only happens once in a lifetime, and it's important to stop and take stock. It's also important to be surrounded by a community that cares during both good times and bad.

Vivian is so excited to leave for Iowa. She thinks it's just the coolest, most glamorous place in the world. You'd think we were headed to Hollywood! Pretty cute.

Jackson generously gave me two kisses today. For that, and so many other reasons, I've finally had a good day!

Planning for Recovery
Monday, May 26, 2008, 9:35 p.m.

A friend of a friend called yesterday to share her experience with breast reconstruction. It sounds arduous. She's been through several procedures in the past year and still isn't done. Hearing the specifics from a survivor is so much more detailed than the basic flyover doctors provide.

At the gym today, I asked a couple of trainers if they've worked out with anyone directly after a hysterectomy. The reason I asked was to find out how long before one can be back to lifting weights. Neither had, but one has worked with a woman who had a lat flap, which is what I'm likely to choose. This procedure takes part of the lat, a.k.a. latissimus dorsi, muscle out of the back, moves it to the pectoral muscle (my pec on the right side is already ruined because of the lumpectomy and radiation), and then attaches an implant to the lat. The woman this trainer worked with isn't having any implants put on; she's just having the muscle moved.

As I was talking with the trainers, I realized they're the ones I'm going to trust to get me back into shape after a mastectomy. The doctors are only responsible for getting a person back to minimal function. They want to make sure I can drive a car, take care of myself, and work. But I want to do so much more than the minimum. For me, going to the gym isn't about getting skinny. It is about getting strong. It's always been important to me to stay strong. Even if they surgically move my muscles around a la Frankenstein, I want to be able to make the muscles I have left as strong as possible.

Although I love working out, the diet part of my fitness regime has been very difficult. I started comfort eating with the diagnosis, and I'm still comfort eating at breakneck speed. I haven't gained any weight lately, just early on, but I can't seem to lose any weight now, either. I was never a person prone to overeating, but now as I seek comfort with food, I can eat so much more than I ever could in the past. I know overeating is bad for my health, but food is providing solace. When I was a little kid, my attitude toward food was that I could take it or leave it. I remember thinking that if they ever invented a pill that could replace food, I'd gladly take it, because eating was such a boring waste of time. But now, I understand the joy and relief that comes along with eating—especially chocolate, cake, and cookies.

When will I be able to eat less and move more? Maybe tomorrow?

Wrapping Up
Wednesday, May 28, 2008, 9:47 p.m.

We're in full prep mode for my hysterectomy on Tuesday. At home, that means staying on top of the laundry, keeping the house picked up, and doing the extra cleaning that needs to be done only every so often. It's great to be super busy.

At work, I'm getting ready by wrapping up and informing my backups of the things they can do to help when I'm out. It's difficult to prepare to leave my job for a few weeks, partly because work is so exciting now. I'd much rather just keep working, which makes it hard to let go. But over-all, I'm ready to have this surgery behind me. I look forward to spending some recovery time outdoors, weather permitting.

Some worry is hovering over this procedure. If they do have to aban-don the laparoscopic surgery in favor of larger incisions, I know it will be a much longer recovery time. Wade and I are also anticipating the stress of waiting a few days for the final pathology report. Hopefully, we'll get word that no cancer was in the ovaries, tubes, or uterus.

Tomorrow is my pre-op exam with my family physician. Later in the afternoon, I'll meet with a plastic surgeon. I'm looking forward to see-ing photos of reconstructive surgery. I've talked with a couple of women who've chosen various reconstructions. At this point, it's still an abstract concept to me. I want to imagine all the possibilities, including going flat.

My spiritual life is still empty. I've decided to seek professional help. I left a voice mail for our priest. He has to be the gentlest soul in the universe and always knows what to say. I know he'll give me some insight before the surgery.

The other night, I dreamed I had published a book. It had become a huge success. I was working on my second book, but the cancer had me-tastasized. I'd been diagnosed as terminal, so I only had a small amount of time left to live. In my dream, I had a dilemma of needing to decide how to spend my time—working at my job or writing?

It got me thinking about the time impoverishment we all suffer from in modern life. I've also been thinking about other writing I'd like to do. I got to thinking about some of the amazing, brave people I've met in support group who are facing metastatic cancer that cannot be cured, and I'm so curious about their stories. Maybe once I'm done telling my story, that would be a meaningful project to pursue.

My darling orange cat, Rocko, is giving me his come-hither look. Oh, how I love to snuggle that little kitty man. Cue the Barry White music.

Plastic Surgeon

Thursday, May 29, 2008, 10:46 p.m.

Wow. What a day—I hardly know where to begin. As anticipated, my pre-op exam was boring. My family doctor reassured me twice that "this is really just a formality." Despite his nonchalance, I couldn't relax all day. This afternoon, Wade and I met with a plastic surgeon. The first thing Dr. Harp said was that one of his patients is willing to talk with me to share her experience. He brought me back to an exam room where she was waiting, introduced us, and left us to talk. She told me about her procedures, and we compared notes on our cancers. Then she showed me her new breasts. They were amazing. They looked totally real. She'd had bilateral mastectomy with lat flaps and implants and recently had her nipples made. Although she didn't have the tattoos for the areolas yet, she still looked great. She was happy with Dr. Harp and pleased with his work. She works in health care, so she knows he's one of the best in town. She explained which aspects had been painful. I asked questions and took notes.

During our conversation, she left her breasts uncovered. I discovered something that most men already know. It's hard to maintain eye contact with a woman sometimes. I wanted to stare at her breasts, because they looked so natural. She did have a long scar on the side of each breast and two smaller ones around the recently created nipple. She also turned around to show me the scars on her back where they removed the lat muscles. While I'm not one to parade around the gym locker room without a towel, I also don't cover myself up at the locker room like a sheepish teenager. But it's still strange to have a full conversation with a topless woman.

Dr. Harp is a darling guy with a crooked little mustache. I love him because he said, "You're too skinny to use your abdominal muscle and fat." I haven't been called "skinny" since third grade, and today I'm twenty-five pounds over my usual comfortable weight. It was fun to hear I'm "too skinny" for anything.

Aside from being flattering, Dr. Harp was informative. He explained why he doesn't believe in using expanders. This is a relief, because they make for many office visits, and they're painful. He showed us photos of his work, but nothing was as helpful as meeting with his patient. Breasts are so three-dimensional that two-dimensional photos don't tell the whole story. I was impressed by the transparency he demonstrated by being willing to let me talk with an existing patient. He even suggested I seek a second opinion and provided me with another doctor's name.

He took a look at my breasts and explained that he wouldn't be able to use the existing skin on my right breast because it has scars from the lumpectomy and from the radiation. He'll use skin from my back instead. He took out a purple marker and drew a shape on my breast that would show how much back skin he'd use to construct the breast. While they won't look as natural as the woman's breasts I saw today (she didn't have radiation), he showed me photos of the result I could expect. When I asked him how long I'd need off work, he quickly replied, "Five weeks." After I expressed shock, he backed down and said that if I wanted to go back to work after two weeks, he wouldn't make me sit out. As long as I didn't need to lift anything heavy, I'd be OK.

He reassured me that I'd have full use of my body after surgery. I was worried that removing muscle from my back might create a lasting disability. He explained that even when construction workers have lat muscles removed—to rebuild legs that are ruined in motorcycle accidents, for example—they can go back to physically demanding work eventually.

I left feeling very reassured and confident that I can do this surgery. It won't be as painful or involved as I'd thought. In addition to the four scars I'll get next week with the hysterectomy and oophorectomy, I can look forward to yet another four scars to add to my collection with the mastectomy and reconstruction. I'm convinced that as the population ages, some day surgical scars will be all the rage.

Then lightning struck. A friend of a friend was diagnosed with breast cancer. This woman is younger than I am, and her youngest child is an infant. I called her, and we had a long conversation about doctors, clinics, genetic testing, and so on. She works in the health care field, so I worry that she won't have the luxury of ignorance that I had going into this whole process. One thing I neglected to tell her is how important it is to allow others to help. Accepting help is difficult, and I imagine that, as a health care professional, she's accustomed to being so capable it may be harder to let others pitch in.

My journey is turning from a marathon into an Ironman. But talking to this newly diagnosed woman today made me realize how much I've grown in the past eight months. I've become a new and improved version of myself. Wade remarked today on my improved self-esteem. Truth be told, I feel more confident than before my diagnosis because everything is now in perspective.

Prayer is coming easily, at last. As I write this, I pray for the newly diagnosed woman and for her husband and family. I pray for doctors and nurses who bear the emotional responsibility of working with patients. I give thanks for the supportive community surrounding my family. I pray that all other patients allow that support in their lives, as well. Amen.

Fancy Soda
Monday, June 2, 2008, 11:13 a.m.

Yesterday, Jackson got his first little time-outs. I was in the kitchen making dinner, Vivian was reading, and Wade was up north fishing. Jackson often takes a running start and crashes into me with a big hug around my legs. But yesterday, for some unknown reason, he decided he should use my legs as a punching bag. His little fists went right, left, right, left, as fast as he could. It was really cute and didn't hurt, but he needs to learn hitting is not OK, so I said, "No hitting!" Then he laughed, backed up, and delivered a kick. "No kicking!" I told him. I redirected him into the other room. Then when I was on the phone a few minutes later, he bit my leg! This was his first bite, and immediately my brain fast-forwarded to him getting kicked out of preschool for biting. Never mind he hasn't started preschool yet. He spent his first time-out in Vivian's room on the bed with the door shut. He hated it and screamed the whole time. I came back one minute later and explained why he got the time-out, told him I love him, and gave him a hug. A few minutes later, he delivered another punch to my leg and got another time-out. This morning, he tried a punch, and I showed him how to set up the pillows on the couch to punch, which he really enjoyed.

After taking Vivian to school and doing a little pillow punching, Jackson and I walked to the pharmacy to pick up my liquid magnesium citrate to "prepare the bowel" for tomorrow's surgery. I chose the lemon flavor, because the other flavor was cherry and bright red. I'm still averse to drinking anything red. In thirty-five minutes, I'll drink my first bottle, and then an hour later, another bottle. Then I'll be housebound, because I can't be too far away from a bathroom. The pharmacist said I should be fine by tonight. I'm only allowed clear liquids today. I wasn't hungry until just around eleven, which surprised me because I've always been a big breakfast eater.

At this moment, I feel OK about the surgery. On Saturday morning, though, I was stressed about it. The house was a mess. I worried about the liquid diet and magnesium citrate. I worried about being in the hospital. If it were happening in the same hospital where I had the kids and my lumpectomy, I'd probably be feeling a bit easier—but it's a different hospital, so I'm just not as sure what to expect. I worried about the recovery at home, looking at my bedroom walls like I did after chemo. Wade reminded me of the differences between surgical recovery and chemo recovery, which relieved me.

While Vivian has said she's not nervous for my surgery, and Jackson is too little to know, I think they're both picking up on my stress and expressing fears about the more concrete things that they can understand. For example, last night, Vivian woke in the middle of the night, dreaming there was a wasp in her room. Little Jackson normally loves hearing garbage trucks and airplanes, but this morning, he was afraid of the sound of both and ran into my arms.

Jackson and my mom just got back from the park, and they're eating lunch. Jackson is explaining to my mom that he's a cookie monster and making lots of noise as he eats his hard-boiled egg. I'm going to enjoy the sights, sounds, and smells of their meal—and then drink my own liquid-laxative lunch. It's in a glass bottle, so I'm going to pretend it's a fancy, expensive soda. Yummy.

The Bare Necessities
Tuesday, June 3, 2008, 9:20 a.m.

OK, I take that back about pretending the magnesium citrate is a fancy soda. I nearly gagged after the first sip, and I had to plug my nose to drink the whole ten ounces. And let's just say it, um, did its job very effectively.

Last night, we spent time drawing tattoos on each other with watercolor pencil. I played the piano, which I haven't done for ages. I played one of my favorite songs from childhood for the kids, "The Bare Necessities" from Disney's *The Jungle Book*. Vivian thought that was a riot, but Jackson couldn't be bothered with it.

I slept great and even slept much of the afternoon. We're all ready to go this morning. Whenever I want to make sure my kids eat a big breakfast, pancakes will do the trick, so that's what I made for them this morning, but my clear-liquid diet meant I couldn't partake.

Last night, Vivian and I walked to the penny-candy store a block away to get some hard candy for me after dinner. My dinner was chicken broth. As we walked, I said, "I'm sorry I can't make it to your writing celebration tomorrow." She started to cry because she didn't connect my surgery with her writing celebration. Luckily, her "aunt" Irene agreed to step in and attend.

Well, time to leave for the hospital. I'm sure Wade will make the next entry for me. Thank you for your kind thoughts and many prayers!

Happy Camper
Tuesday, June 3, 2008, 9:58 p.m.

It's Wade, the husband, writing here. Good evening to all the cancer-fighting storm troopers. Why storm troopers, you ask? I'll get to that.

Camille and I had a great morning today, as weird as that may sound, joking, laughing, and being a general nuisance to some of the staff in the pre-op exam room. We were (oddly enough) excited to get the procedure over with so we could process all our good news, or just news, or even bad news, the results didn't seem to matter as much as laughing together and knowing that we'd have some sort of closure by the end of the day. Some breathing room, if you will.

I tried to be a good employee and wake up early to get at least a couple of hours of work done before the surgery, but when the birds woke me at 5:15, the thought of pancakes with the family convinced me to stay in bed just a while longer. I'm glad I stayed to see Vivian off to school (face paint and all) and to give Jackson a "squeezer" before taking Camille to the hospital. I'm so glad Camille's mom is able to watch Jackson; it's a relief to have him with his grandma through all of this.

I just want to take a minute here and say our hospital is great. Where else can you start an operation forty-five minutes *early*? Not to mention the constant updates from the operating room delivered by a sweet little Swedish grandma with her *Fargo*-esque accent. They updated me about every fifteen to twenty minutes about where the doctor was in the procedure. What a relief.

As I sat in the waiting lounge, getting my updates, I noticed that the doctors were giving the "that sums it up" speeches to the families after finishing their respective operations. These updates were given in the lounge, not in a separate room that would afford some notion of privacy. So when the sweet Swedish grandma asked me to follow her to a post-op consultation room, needless to say, my heart sank. Immediately, I suspected the worst, but then Dr. Beckman came in with a great smile on her face and informed me that there were no tumors, growths, or abnormalities of any kind. In fact, all had gone swimmingly.

I thought I'd retch then and there.

I told her about my observations in the lounge and that I was worried about the need for a consultation room, and she laughed and said that she thought it odd that some doctors do that—that it seems a bit uncouth and that she prefers the privacy of the consultation rooms. I have to say, I absolutely agree. I heard things today about people's conditions that broke my heart, made me sick, and sometimes made me feel dirty for overhearing what was being said. I guess that a surgical waiting room is a place where you can definitely find cohorts in misery, pain, and celebration. How very odd.

Camille is doing great. Minor pain, kinda loopy, pretty sleepy—overall, she's a happy camper. She should be home tomorrow afternoon sometime, provided she's still well in the morning. We were laughing again this evening when she was arguing (somewhat slurred with pain meds) with the food service people because she wanted a grilled cheese sandwich *and* cheese pizza. They said she could only have one. OK. She could have *two* grilled cheese sandwiches or *two* cheese pizzas, but not one of each. It was really, really funny. Both of the nurses in her room at the time were crying from laughter as I shook my head in the corner.

2 cheese pizzas: $450.

2 grilled cheese sandwiches: $437.

1 bowl tepid tomato soup: $250.

Bringing your nurses to tears with laughter: priceless.

Wade

Storm Troopers
Thursday, June 5, 2008, 5:14 p.m.

I just read Wade's update from Tuesday. It was pretty funny when the food-service people wouldn't do my bidding. Wade mentioned storm troopers but didn't explain why. It's because, as I did after my lumpectomy, I got to wear the storm-trooper boots on my legs to prevent blood clots. They're pretty cool because they puff up and give you a leg massage every few minutes. Some people don't like them, but I love them.

The surgery was over in just forty-five minutes, when it could have gone for ninety. I was so calm waiting for the surgery, I didn't even need the sedation before the operating room; I went in without any drugs until they were ready to start the operation. The time in the hospital wasn't so bad. I had some pain when I'd move, and the narcotics gave me a strange reaction. When Wade left on Tuesday night, I kind of freaked out and called him to come back because I was afraid to be alone. I couldn't explain why. Then two girlfriends, Irene and Alison, came over, and we had a great chat.

When I was still in the hospital, a nurse from integrative care stopped by and showed me some natural pain-relief techniques. She demonstrated how to use my hand to "sponge" away the pain wherever I'm feeling it. Last night, I was having some pain, and it worked just great. The only place it hurts is at the very bottom of my belly at the larger incision site. Starting to move again was tricky in the hospital. The main nurse I had last night takes yoga classes, and she reminded me to move on the exhale, which made a big difference in comfortably getting in and out of bed.

This is the first time that I've had an all-female care team, and I loved it. I felt nurtured and not condescended to at all. They all really seemed to have my recovery as their top priority. Dr. Beckman explained that over the next few days, I'll have even more intense menopause symptoms. Last night, I had night sweats and had to change my T-shirt. My tummy is still puffed up from the carbon dioxide they use to inflate my abdomen during the laparoscopic surgery. It will be a week before my tummy deflates. I don't have many clothes that fit this new puffy torso, so it will be sweatpants for the next week, I suppose.

Last night and today while I was resting, Dr. Rocko was sitting right by my belly purring. That little kitty man delivers such wonderful medicine. This morning, I walked Vivian to her last day of school, which has her feeling mixed emotions.

This morning, I was still taking Percocet, and it was making me feel really stoned. Now I'm just on Tylenol and Motrin. The pain is managed with those, so I finally have my mind back. I hate the feeling of a narcotic stupor. Tonight, Wade and the kids are eating at a friend's house so I can rest. It's storming outside, and I have a copy of Agatha Christie's *Murder on the Orient Express* to read, which is a perfect fit for the weather.

Hooray!
Friday, June 6, 2008, 4:47 p.m.

Just got the best phone call. My pathology report came back, and everything is negative. Not even one microscopic speck of cancer!!! Hooray! Vivian is coming back from her yoga class in a few minutes; I have a big plate of chocolate-chip cookies for her and a full weekend ahead of us to rest and enjoy.

I wish I could go back to work on Monday, but I know it's too soon. I'm still a little out of it. But I'm totally off the narcotics and am having no pain, so I'm free to start driving my car again. Maybe Wade and I can go to the movies this weekend. It's been so long since we've done that, and there's a new movie I can't wait to see.

Last night was lovely with the thunder, lightning, and *Murder on the Orient Express*. I hope for more storms tonight.

Just before I got the "good news, no cancer" phone call, I was paying bills and starting to get a little stressed about the cash flow. (We have plenty. It's just tight because I have an extra two-week wait between commission checks this month.) But after getting that phone call, I realized I was sweating the small stuff, and who needs that?

Summertime

Monday, June 9, 2008, 7:35 p.m.

Today has been one of those carefree, relaxing summer days. The weather is perfect, and I just returned to a (fairly) clean home after hanging out with the neighbors. We have so few months of nice weather in Minnesota. So during the summer, everyone lives outdoors, and impromptu gatherings are common.

The universe is shining on me in so many ways today. My book group sent a gift certificate for a cool clothing catalog. Plus, a cousin sent a Target gift card just in time for us to realize Jackson will soon be ready for the next size up in car seats!

I'm still puffed up like a balloon from the carbon dioxide during surgery. Unlike gaining a few pounds on vacation and still being able to cram the extra fat into your jeans, this puffy belly of mine is all air, so it's rock hard. I look five months pregnant, but the bump goes all the way up to my diaphragm. Gym pants are the only ones that fit. I have two skirts with elastic waists, so I can wear those, as well. I'm thinking of starting a website called something like Dressing Despite Disease, where people can post tips to look decent despite various fashion challenges—being puffed up with CO_2, wearing a sports bra for weeks during radiation, having drainage tubes hanging out after lumpectomy or mastectomy. There must be other medical conditions that create fashion disasters. Maybe there's a good resource out there already?

Stitches

Father's Day, Sunday, June 15, 2008, 9:52 p.m.

Today was another beautiful day. Wade went fishing with a friend this morning and was scolded by Vivian this afternoon, "You should want to spend time with your family on Father's Day!" Someday she'll understand that Dad going fishing can be the best Father's Day gift.

Last week, I went to work for a few hours each day and felt fine. It was good to feel like I was having "bonus" time at work. It was enjoyable and productive, but very tiring. On Tuesday, I slept in until 10:30 after going to work for just two hours on Monday! It's hard to believe how easily I get worn out. The only pain I have is when I'm done going to the bathroom, my belly cramps up. When I told Wade about it, he said the surgeon said that would happen for a while as my bladder gets used to its new place. Rather than starting pain meds, I've been doing deep breathing as I sit on the pot. Wouldn't my yoga teacher be proud?!

On Thursday, the stitches were removed. It was quick and painless. Later that night, I felt something in my belly button (that's where one of the four incisions was) and pulled out a piece of monofilament (like a thin fishing line used for stitches) that had fallen in after she cut my stitches out. I thought I maybe felt something else but ignored it. Then on Saturday night, I was sure I could feel something in there. Wade took a look, and sure enough, one stitch was remaining. He tried to get it out, but couldn't, so I'll have to go back in to have it removed this week.

Yesterday, a member of our church prayer chain stopped by with a gift. The prayer chain members each wrote a prayer for me, and they bound it into a lovely book. The prayers are beautiful.

Wade, Jackson, and Vivian are all sleeping, so I'd best join them. I plan to go to work tomorrow.

Bad Haircut

Thursday, June 19, 2008, 9:36 p.m.

Vivian was a real little angel today. She's making pink breast cancer hope ribbons and origami flowers for a Susan G. Komen lemonade stand fund-raiser. She's wanted to raise money for breast cancer since my diagnosis. Today, she taught me how to make origami flowers and worked with me on the ribbons.

When I told her I needed to write tonight, she wanted me to mention that her behavior has been fantastic lately, which is true. Just one example is her haircut yesterday. We've been working hard to curb our expenses because we have a vacation just around the corner. We decided I should go back to cutting the kids' hair myself. I have no real talent for it, but Vivian's cut is pretty simple. Then she decided she wanted bangs. I took the scissors and was aiming for the bangs to fall at her eyebrows, but somehow cut them a full inch above the middle of her forehead! Immediately, I could see that it looked like she'd cut her own hair. I worked out a solution where she can slick back her bangs and use a barrette until they grow out. I felt so bad that I gave her ten dollars to buy new barrettes. She cried for a few minutes but was very quick to forgive my mistake. She's even willing to let me cut her hair again. What a resilient little lady.

The plans for my final surgery (mastectomy and reconstruction) are starting to fall into place. August seems like the best time based on my work and social schedule. It's nice to have the luxury of time to plan this surgery.

Lemonade Stand

Saturday, June 21, 2008, 9:56 p.m.

The weather was perfect today for Vivian's lemonade stand fund-raiser. She raised $521 for Susan G. Komen for the Cure! The lemonade sold out. One of Vivian's classmates also did a lemonade stand to raise money for breast cancer. Our two families took the kids to Dairy Queen after all their hard work to celebrate. This first-grade friend and Vivian have been talking about having a fair to raise money for breast cancer all year. During our ice-cream adventure, I commented, "You both did so well with your lemonade stands, you won't even have to do a fair now."

Both kids looked at me and said, "Oh no, we're still going to have the fair."

As parents, we weren't sure what to say, so we started to help them plan a fair to raise money! The generous nature of Vivian and her class-mate astound me.

Insomnia

Friday, June 27, 2008, 4:24 a.m.

My insomnia has reached an all-time high. All my life, I've had insom-nia. As a seven-year-old, I recall trying to fall asleep at slumber par-ties, listening enviously as my friends breathing changed from sleepy to asleep. Tonight, I haven't been able to fall asleep at all. It's 4:30 a.m. now. Some crazy birds started singing an hour ago. I've abandoned all hope for sleep today.

Starting in the hospital three weeks ago, I've been taking lorazepam (the generic version of Ativan, an antianxiety pill) nearly every night. It's the same drug that allowed me to rest during chemo. Just one week ago, a lorazepam would bring near instant relaxation to my body and mind. As of Monday, the effectiveness of the drug has dwindled. Tonight, it isn't working at all. I'm afraid to take a double dose. Tomorrow, I'll invest in some sleeping pills. Normally, I hate to add more chemicals to the mix, but I really need to sleep.

In addition to suffering from insomnia, I'm suffering from envy. Big time. Over stupid things. Talking to another cancer survivor today, she explained that her "percentage" (shorthand for her chances of surviving five years without cancer recurrence) is 90 percent without even doing chemo. I had to do surgery, chemo, and radiation just to get to 70 per-cent. Of course, I'm happy that her prognosis is so good, but why can't

I have that too? Why did this have to happen in the first place? Why am I asking these questions now? I suspect it's because I'm not preparing for a surgery, or a chemo, or a radiation treatment—and I'm not recovering from surgery, chemo, or radiation. It's this in-between time when I feel fairly healthy and don't have an immediate challenge in front of me that the emotions bubble up to the surface.

Hair envy is my other affliction at the moment. The novelty of a hip, short cut has completely faded for me. At a baseball game the other night, a woman with long, pretty brunette hair stood near us for part of the game. I tried not to stare at her, but I just wanted to gaze at her beautiful hair. I was so wishing for my long, pretty brunette hair. It will literally take years for it to grow back down to my elbows, where it was before chemo. How could I be so calm about losing my hair only to feel so envious now that it's finally starting to grow back? Anyone who has ever grown out bangs knows how frustrating it is to have in-progress hair.

At a business luncheon this week, I approached a group of three strangers, and we made introductions. One looked at the work ID hanging from my lanyard and saw a photo of a woman with long, dark brown hair. She looked back up at me and remarked, "You have a whole new look since your photo!"

I simply said, "It's true!"

Another woman commented, "A major summer haircut."

I replied truthfully, "It's that and much more." Then I steered the conversation back to the luncheon we were about to attend.

In professional settings, unless it's someone I connect with on a personal level, there just isn't time to discuss the whole health issue. One client hadn't seen me in a year and remarked when she saw me, "Wow, massive makeover!"

I replied with an enthusiastic, "Yes, it sure is!" and that was the end of it.

Each situation is different. For the most part, I'm totally comfortable discussing my health. I even hope to become a resource to help others. But so often when meeting new people, there just isn't time for the whole conversation.

Dr. Rocko is giving me his lovey-dovey eyes and purring. He thinks he can seduce me into sleep, but I'm afraid even a perfect kitty man can't help me sleep right now.

Menopause
Sunday, June 29, 2008, 9:19 p.m.

Finally, sleep found me at 6:00 a.m. on Friday. Then Vivian found me at 7:30 a.m., ready for breakfast. The day turned out to be OK, considering I'd had so little sleep. The nurse at my surgeon's office said the insomnia is due to menopause. I can expect it to continue for at least the next six months. She said it tends to come and go. Over-the-counter sleeping pills are safe, and she's going to send me a prescription for something stronger, just in case. Turns out the over-the-counter Unisom was plenty. It gave me a good night's sleep on Friday and Saturday. But today, I felt exhausted and out of it. In a little while, I'm going to try sleeping on my own, but I'm nervous I'll need a sleeping pill.

The nurse also mentioned that I can expect to feel moody thanks to menopause. While menopause technically started during chemo, the hysterectomy and oophorectomy were the final nails in the menopausal coffin, so to speak. As a result, the menopause symptoms of night sweats, hot flashes, moodiness, and insomnia are more dramatic. Both yesterday and today, I found myself snapping at the kids over nothing. I felt furious with Wade as he cleaned the kitchen, which I know is insane—a wife furious with a kitchen-cleaning husband!

Cured?
Saturday, July 5, 2008, 1:23 p.m.

Sleep has been much easier this week. Thank goodness. We had a blast at the Fourth of July barbecue and fireworks with friends. We're on our way to another barbecue tonight.

I'm on a once-every-three-months appointment schedule with my oncologist, Dr. Anderson. Thankfully, my blood tests showed nothing has metastasized. That's the news we'll want every three months from now on. If my blood tests look suspicious, then CT scans, MRIs, and so on will follow. At my last appointment, I asked if I should also be on the lookout for any symptoms of metastasizing. He said no, but I must tell him if I notice something out of the ordinary that has no other explanation.

If I tell him I have a backache, he needs to check it out with tests. But if there's a reasonable explanation (I overdid it lifting the kids), then I don't need to tell him. If something lasts for two weeks without an explanation, then he needs to know. He has some patients that are constantly reporting trouble, thus they're constantly having tests.

I also asked him to review my original staging. By staging, I mean when he told me that I'm Stage III, indicating the tumors were big and the cancer had spread to my lymph nodes. When he first told me I was Stage III, he said the odds of making it five years without the cancer spreading are 70 percent after chemo, surgery, and radiation. So I asked him about that statistic in detail—at what point am I officially cured? He didn't really have an answer. I was starting to cry and was so glad Wade is attending my appointments with me. Dr. Anderson said, yes, I do have more than a 50 percent chance of the cancer staying gone. But five years isn't a magic number. Cancer can come back in ten or fifteen years or more. There are no guarantees in life. I know that, but it still made me cry. At times, I feel so sad and worried. I asked again, as I did a few months ago, if I could live to be an old lady, and he said yes. At this point, having that hope is a gift.

He did have some concrete bad news for me. I'd forgotten all about the DXA bone scan I had a few months ago. It revealed that I have osteopenia, which means low bone density. It's the precursor to osteoporosis. This was one of Dr. Anderson's concerns in determining if I need tamoxifen or an aromatase inhibitor to block the remaining estrogen in my body. It's my lower back and hips that show the osteopenia. Because I'm only thirty-eight, his concern is that if I stay on the aromatase inhibitor, I could start having fractures by age fifty, so he's switching me to tamoxifen.

This isn't a big deal, except that I have to call him before taking any new medications. Even ibuprofen can interfere with it. I'm also bummed out because I need to switch antidepressants because my current antidepressant will interact with the tamoxifen.

Many years ago, during a rough patch in my life, my family physician gave me the antidepressant Lexapro, and I found that not only did it help with the tough situation I was in at that time, it also made me feel better than ever. It improved my mental clarity. It reduced my levels of worry and anxiety, which I didn't realize were constant until they went away. For that reason, I've stayed on the Lexapro even after the difficult situation resolved. The idea of switching to another antidepressant makes me nervous. I hope it has the same benefits. The new antidepressant they're recommending will have the added benefit of reducing hot flashes, which are more annoying than disruptive at this point.

Now that I have cancer, everyone tells me about any cancer diagnosis they hear about. Just last night, I heard about another woman being diagnosed—with lung cancer that has metastasized. She has a CaringBridge site, so I went on it to tell her about some of the helpful resources available. It's awful to hear of a new diagnosis, but it's a blessing to share what I've learned. I can't wait for the day that this entire disease is extinct.

Vacation Nails

Tuesday, July 15, 2008, 9:33 p.m.

We just returned from a family vacation to Northern Minnesota, which was very relaxing. It was a working vacation for Wade, as he successfully potty-trained Jackson! Now that we're back, Jackson isn't so interested in the potty, but at least during vacation, he experienced the potty joy. He also was a wild man at the water park we visited.

Vivian loves the outdoors, so hiking, bouldering, and rock climbing were her favorite vacation activities. I enjoyed identifying wild flowers with a new field guide. Having a full week away from television and computers gave us all the opportunity to reconnect with a simpler world.

Vivian and I put cute little flower decals on our fingernails and enjoyed our silly vacation nails.

During the time off, I had too much time to think. I spent quite a bit of vacation time worrying about the future—more specifically, about the cancer metastasizing. It's time for me to let those thoughts go and spend time being busy once again at work, away from sad thoughts. There's no point in worry because it won't help anything. So the cute vacation nail polish is coming off so I can focus once more on work and distraction.

Today, I found out that my father is responsible for passing along the BRCA2 mutation to me. We know for sure because my mother had the BRCA2 genetic test, which showed that she doesn't carry the mutation. I called one of my paternal cousins to share the news, and I felt so bad telling her about it. On the one hand, it's good information to know. Hopefully, their mother (my dad's sister) didn't inherit the gene, which would mean they're all clear. However, it does mean they'll need to decide about testing, increased surveillance (mammograms, etc.), and discussions with their doctors and children. This journey just seems to keep dragging along with so many additional tasks; it can be depressing. I'll be sending out the VD letter my genetic counselor drafted in the next few days.

Jackson is now on my lap wanting to help type, so that's my cue to shut down for tonight.

Hello, Lymphedema

Monday, July 21, 2008, 10:11 p.m.

I had a quite a scare last Friday. A few days earlier, I bumped my hand on my file cabinet and thought nothing of it. On Friday morning, I noticed my right hand was a bit swollen. By that afternoon, it had really puffed up, so I called my lymphedema clinic. The therapist said to get some antibiotics right away and to put on my compression sleeve and glove. Oops, I never got a compression sleeve and glove, because this wasn't supposed to happen to me! After the phone conversation, I was hysterical, calling Wade, crying my eyes out. The remainder of the afternoon was spent calling my doctor to get antibiotics to prevent infection and getting my compression garments from the lymphedema clinic.

I spent some time at the lymphedema clinic checking out a catalog for women who decide not to get reconstructed after mastectomy. I tried to have an open mind, but going flat still doesn't seem like the right option for me.

As the compression fitter showed me how to put on the sleeve and glove, I noticed that even though it's made to be flesh colored, nobody has flesh that color. When I left wearing my sleeve and glove, I felt embarrassed, like a dog wearing an Elizabethan-collar cone around its neck to prevent it from licking a wound. It occurred to me that I couldn't possibly get much more attractive—those extra pounds from my post-diagnosis comfort eating, my one-inch crop of hair, and now a lovely "flesh-colored" sleeve. If only I could grow a big pimple on the end of my nose, the look would be complete.

Wade says the sleeve isn't that noticeable. I wore it all day Friday, Saturday, and Sunday. I meant to wear it today, but somehow it got lost between the dryer and my bedroom this morning. As a result, I arrived late to work, only to find my computer didn't want to cooperate. The day seemed a bust until evening, when we decided to go to a little indoor water park with the neighbors. My neighbor's friend brought his friend along, who happens to be a famous Hollywood actress. She had lovely, long blonde hair, and I felt like such a schlepper in nearly nonexistent hair and my mommy swimsuit. But she was very nice, Jackson had a blast, Vivian was happy to be swimming with her little neighbor friend, so who cares what I look like?

My hand that was so swollen looks almost totally normal tonight, and I'm seeing my lymphedema therapist on Wednesday. That same day, I'll meet with arguably the best plastic surgeon in town for a second opinion. After this meeting, I should be able to schedule my very last procedure, the mastectomy. I can't wait to have it all behind me.

Waiting for Mastectomy

Wednesday, July 23, 2008, 10:11 p.m.

Today was one of the most difficult days so far. Don't even know where to begin. The good news is that I found Dr. Nicholson, the plastic surgeon of my dreams. He came complete with a Minnesota Wild wristwatch. The bad news is that he wants me to be six months out from radiation before we do surgery. That pushes it to the end of October or early November. My hopes of having the procedure at the end of the summer are dashed. The time frame I wanted would have worked on so many levels. I would have missed the State Fair, but not much else.

Dr. Nicholson operates at the hospital of my choice, plus his team includes a lymphedema doctor. His office is more like a spa. When we arrived, the nurse offered us drinks, which is very unlike a typical clinic. My water came in an actual glass with ice. Wade's coffee was served in a fancy teacup with a matching saucer.

Despite the amenities, Dr. Nicholson delivered the bad news that he wants to use expanders, which means one surgery with a long recovery time, one outpatient procedure six months later, and several office visits for saline to be added to the expanders in between. Ultimately, I should get a better result, but ugh. Luckily, he only wants to take muscle from the right lat muscle in my back, which will decrease the pain and chances of complications compared with taking both the right and left lat.

Today, I was feeling very depressed after the meeting with Dr. Nicholson. My mind was set on an end-of-summer surgery, but now I'll have to wait until winter. Moving forward with all these procedures has been empowering, plus it's kept me busy. We also wanted to get everything done in this calendar year because we've already paid our $3,000 in out-of-pocket expenses for the year. Looks like next year will be another $3,000. Cancer is expensive.

I was depressed about waiting for the surgery when I realized how ridiculous my life has become. I'm bummed out because I can't get my boobs chopped off next month? Come on, that's a crazy reason to be depressed. That thought made me feel a little better, because at least I could laugh at how ridiculous things have become. Wade also reminded me that menopause can cause mood swings. Then I remembered that stress is cumulative. All the stress of the last ten months has been offset by action. Now the action is slowing, leaving more time for it all to sink in.

One of Wade's buddies stopped by tonight, so I'm going to hang out and chat with them. Surely they'll tell me some dirty jokes to get my mind off my breasts!

Strange Dream
Monday, July 28, 2008, 9:46 p.m.

Last night, I had a strange dream. Vivian was seven, the same age she is in real life. We found out that she was pregnant! If that wasn't weird enough, in the dream, the most upsetting part was that I didn't even get to tell her about the bird and the bees. When I woke up, it dawned on me that the dream was about me worrying about postponing the surgery, thus postponing telling Vivian about the mastectomy. I want to tell her that it's coming up because I'm afraid she'll overhear a conversation and I won't be the one to tell her. The counselors have recommended waiting until we have the details of when surgery will take place, but I think now is the time to tell her. I asked her how my last surgery was for her, and she said it was hard having me in the hospital and not being able to spend time with me. Hopefully, I'll soon find a way to tell her about this next surgery.

My right-hand lymphedema stopped swelling, only to start again a few days later. I'm wearing the compression sleeve, but the swelling is getting a little worse each day. Tomorrow, I'll see the lymphedema therapist, and I'll need to go back twice a week for at least three weeks. It's not clear if they can get my arm back to the original size. The swelling is minor, only two to three centimeters larger than the other arm, so it's not too noticeable. But without the compression garments, my arm hurts. I'm trying not to worry about it, but I hate the thought of having to wear this sleeve forever, which is a possibility.

Roller Derby

Wednesday, July 30, 2008, 6:00 p.m.

Remember the lymphedema compression garment I was embarrassed to wear? And how I felt like a dog wearing an Elizabethan collar? Well, the Elizabethan collar has been upgraded to something even more humiliating. Yesterday at the lymphedema therapist, I expected a light massage on my arm to get the lymph fluid moving. I was surprised when she started taking about "wrapping" and "bandaging" with another therapist. At the end of my massage, she proceeded to wrap my arm mummy-style with no less than seven rolls of various bandaging material. The result is what appears to be a broken arm.

After returning to my office, I solicited creative lies from each person who asked, "What happened to your arm?" Suggestions included tennis, rock climbing, and a bad fall. The winner hands down was roller derby. I tested it on a coworker today:

COWORKER. What happened to you?!
ME. Amateur night at the roller derby. Seemed like a good idea at the time.
COWORKER. (*Blank stare.*)
ME. (*Satisfaction that I'd elevated my image to a daring and cool risk-taker while avoiding the very complicated true story.*)

In a few minutes, I'll leave to work out at the gym, where I pray someone else asks what happened to my arm.

Truth be told, the wrapping is much more comfortable than the compression garment. However, sleep was miserable last night because I couldn't stay comfortable with this huge thing on my arm. It can't get wet, so taking a shower involved a plastic garbage bag and one of Vivian's hair bands to keep the bandages dry. Very inconvenient.

Thirty-Nine

Tuesday, August 5, 2008, 4:06 a.m.

Today, I turn thirty-nine. Birthdays have always felt like a personal New Year's Day to me—a time for reflection to take stock of the past year's accomplishments, say good-bye to the old, and look forward to the new. This year feels much different. The accomplishment of my thirty-eighth year was merely surviving it. Never before has there been quite so much to reflect upon.

This past week, I've been wrestling with depression. Work has lost its luster for me. It feels boring and dull. Wade reminded me that we all have times like that with work, but I'm sad because work has been such a great friend and respite from illness during the past year. I'm trying to look at these feelings about being bored with work as natural and as a good sign that life is returning to "normal." However, I miss the urgency and passion I felt for work even a few weeks ago. Writing isn't holding my interest like it has since starting this blog, either. At home, I'm longing for time alone, which is such a luxury in a household with two kids. In my heart, I feel a heavy sadness quite often. On the outside, I'm hating my wrapped, compressed, often painful arm. Lymphedema sucks. I've been trying to home color my two inches of hair to a pretty platinum blonde; instead, it's an unnatural strawberry yellow. This weekend, I'll keep working the bleach to get it right. Why can't I just pay the sixty dollars to get it done in a salon? Maybe in my thirty-ninth year, I can stop being such a cheapskate.

Perhaps birthdays can be tough because we're meant to be happy on them. When life doesn't meet our expectations, it becomes increasingly difficult to be happy. Aimee Mann has a song, "Thirty One Today," in which she writes, "I thought my life would be different somehow, I thought my life would be better by now," which sums up how most of us feel at some points in our lives. My twentysomething self would have expected so much more of my life by now. But of course, as life unfolds, expectations shift, and the real world offers its own surprising twists.

Lately, I've been longing to read about Buddhism because that philosophy appeals to me. One of the key tenets is turning away from attachment. The expectations of my life and what it "should" be is an attachment causing suffering today.

As I let go of my thirty-eighth year, I leave with the knowledge that community surrounds me. I know that if only we ask, people are there to support us.

Part of the sadness I feel today is likely because I can't help but think that on my last birthday, my life was free of the knowledge of cancer. I'd yet to even schedule the first doctor appointment that threw my life into such chaos. The things I miss about my past life are very real, and I'm OK with missing those things. As the beauty of youth fades, the beauty of wisdom emerges, right?

Tonight, we'll go as a family to a butterfly exhibit at the zoo. It will be an appropriate activity for my birthday—the butterflies symbolize new life and, for me, a new year.

Butterflies

Wednesday, August 6, 2008, 10:44 p.m.

My lymphedema therapist said I have an 80 percent chance of getting my arm back to normal size (compared with an 85 percent chance of getting a new breast cancer based on my BRCA2 status—yikes). I'm pulling for the 80 percent chance of getting rid of my lymphedema but hoping against the 85 percent chance that I'll get a new breast cancer.

The butterfly exhibit yesterday was amazing. We could hear their wings beating. So many beautiful exotic species were there. The kids loved it. We had a nice dinner and a walk by a lake, and by the end of the night, I felt like my old self again. My energy has returned, and today turned out to be a good day too. Seems like my perspective has shifted to a better place.

Hair Success

Sunday, August 17, 2008, 10:46 p.m.

Hair success at last! I finally went to a salon for the final bleach and toner, which pulled out the yellow, leaving the pale white / platinum blonde I'd been seeking. That very day, I was at a stoplight applying lipstick, and a young man shouted out, "You're so pretty, you don't need any makeup!" It cracked me up. Having the hair I want makes me feel so much better. I'll keep it blonde and grow out the dark roots, which will look cool, and then after it's just blonde tips, I'll become brunette again. Wade is anxious for me to be brunette again, but he'll have to wait a bit longer; I'm having fun being a blonde.

My right arm is still bandaged, but my arm itself is only one centimeter larger than the left. It's been so frustrating lately because everything takes longer with the bandaging. Typing is uncomfortable and slow. I've been spending about thirty minutes a day bandaging, washing the bandages, and doing physical therapy exercises. I'm hopeful that within two weeks, my arm will be back to normal. It will be nice to not have this constant visible reminder of cancer. I think that's a big part of why my family wants me to be brunette again—it's another visible reminder of the cancer. I'll look more like my old self when I go back to brunette, but for now, being platinum blonde is my "screw you" to cancer.

Lately, I've been having trouble feeling motivated to do much around the house. Wade has even noticed that I'm uncharacteristically lazy. I wonder if it's medication related. The new meds I'm on have made me nauseated and dizzy at times, which are two of the possible side effects listed. Hopefully, it's only temporary.

Memory Issues

Tuesday, September 2, 2008, 8:39 p.m.

First day of school today. Vivian cried when I left her classroom. She has some separation anxiety, which started earlier this summer. Her teacher told me she was fine two minutes after I'd left. Wade thinks on some subconscious level, Vivian is still afraid of losing me.

These days, I'm a bit afraid of losing me too. I worry about the cancer metastasizing. And I don't feel like myself. Wade confirms that I've been confused and irritable. It's not so obvious that other people might notice, but I notice, and Wade does. I'm mostly confused about the days of the week. For example, last Wednesday, I had physical therapy. She gave me enough of the specialty tape to last through two wrappings. On Thursday night, I removed the tape thinking it was already Saturday. Now I'm out of tape and need to go tomorrow morning to pick up more at the clinic. I've also mixed up the dates of Vivian's book group and one client appointment. Yesterday, which was Monday, I thought we'd just returned from our Labor Day weekend trip to Iowa, while we actually returned on Sunday. These bits of confusion really bother me because normally I'm so on the ball with everything. Wade said, "You're just becoming one of us," meaning a normal person, which was very sweet. I moved up my next oncology appointment a full month to Thursday. I'm going to talk about my symptoms, and maybe Dr. Anderson will have some ideas on what's causing my confusion—stress, menopause, my antidepressant, or chemo.

Planning for Vivian's Kids Play for a Cure, Vivian's fund-raising fair is wrapping up. We just have a few more details to wrangle before this Saturday! Truth be told, I've had a blast planning this, and I love having something that Vivian and I can share being excited about.

My arm is still giving me trouble—no pain, but it's still swollen. I met someone today who just gave up on all the lymphedema wrapping. Now she has one arm she calls her "fat arm." After six weeks of working on my arm, I can see how that's tempting. But I'm not ready to give up yet.

Final Plans for Kids Play for a Cure

Friday, September 5, 2008, 10:28 p.m.

The countdown to Kids Play for a Cure is on! I've spent the last two days blissfully planning the final details. The weather looks like it should be perfect. If there's one thing this whole journey has taught me, it's that a life without service is a life that isn't worth living. During my darkest times, I've thought about what's really important: Making the world a better place.

Despite feeling so happy about the Kid's Play fair over the last two days, I'm feeling blue right now. A bunch of neighbors were outside chatting, and I had to go inside to wrap up my stupid arm and massage my faulty lymph nodes. It's not my style to feel sorry for myself, but it's just hard to look on the bright side sometimes.

All of the kids are so excited for tomorrow, and that will need to sustain me. Vivian wants to help with three different activities—making God's Eyes (a yarn-and-Popsicle-stick craft she loves), working behind the sheet of the fishing pond, and making popcorn. I love that she wants to make a difference. I just wish she didn't have a 50 percent chance of having the same rotten gene that got me into this fine mess. I'm crying now, thinking that the money she raises tomorrow may or may not save her own life someday.

Kids Play for a Cure

Sunday, September 7, 2008, 5:23 p.m.

Kids Play for a Cure was a tremendous success. A total of $1,305 has been donated—$435 each to Susan G. Komen, the American Cancer Society, and the Angel Foundation of Minnesota.

We estimate that more than three hundred children came to play with us. Vivian was really running the show while my mom was running after Jackson! The inflatable jumper, face painting, hair wrapping, fish pond, and musical instrument petting zoo were the biggest hits. Many local businesses helped out, so we kept the total expenses low.

Finally being able to give back is such a great feeling. When a television reporter covering the event asked, "How proud are you of your daughter?" I started to cry and said I was bursting with pride. Vivian is an amazing little girl.

Young Barbie

Wednesday, September 10, 2008, 6:43 a.m.

"You look like a brunette Barbie doll," a new friend told me in eighth grade. She was, no doubt, referring to my thick brown hair, which reached nearly to my waist. My face was fringed with bangs that curled perfectly under, just like Barbie's. I was at a new school and reinventing myself.

This fall, twenty-five years after that middle school reinvention, I realize that I've done it again, more dramatically than ever before. While many of the changes marking this reinvention haven't been of my choosing—many others have been. As I look back on that young "Barbie," I wonder what I still have in common with that girl. What she stood for—optimism, youth, hope—seems to have vanished. Just in terms of appearance, I look nothing like a brunette Barbie. With my short, platinum hair, I kind of resemble a Barbie that's had a vicious haircut by a four-year-old. To be fair to my existing do, I have received compliments, including, "It's very Old Hollywood" and "You look like Jean Seberg."

Today, we'll take a huge leap of faith. We close on a new mortgage that will double our existing loan and double the existing square footage of our home. It will allow my mom to move into the mother-in-law apartment we're adding as part of the remodel. We've been wanting her to move in for so long. It's a leap of faith because signing this mortgage assumes we'll be earning more money in the future. For someone unable to work much of the past year, that takes a lot of optimism. Maybe there's more of that eighth-grade brunette Barbie optimism left in me than I'd realized.

Professional Patient

Saturday, September 13, 2008, 12:51 p.m.

You know how professional NASCAR racers get sponsors and put logos all over their cars? Lately, I've been going to so many doctor and physical therapy appointments that I've been thinking about contacting some drug companies to solicit sponsorships in exchange for covering my clothes with their logos. I guess that means I'm starting to feel like I'm a professional patient. It's in this context that I had a come-to-Jesus meeting with myself. I've been complaining and feeling sorry for myself so much lately. Yesterday, I remembered that having gloomy feelings is natural, but how long I stay in those gloomy places is my choice. I also had a conversation with a fellow survivor. Her strength and positivity made me realize I can make a choice to stay in a place of gratitude, moving away from self-pity.

This new resolve was tested yesterday by spending about two hours on the phone with my insurance company and clinics. Rather than feeling sorry for myself that I have to manage all this red tape, I kept reminding myself that it's a good thing to have health insurance and to access clinics. What is it—something like 40 percent?—of people in the United States don't even have health insurance? So I'm reminding myself that these are high-class problems to have, and quit whining.

I've been so distracted at work, unable to get the things done that I demand of myself. Thank heaven I have bosses who understand this doesn't mean I'm permanently checked out. An employment attorney told me a story of a woman telling her boss that she had cancer, to which he replied, "You must be wanting to take some time off work, so you're fired." I'm grateful I have a boss who not only upholds the law but supports me on a personal level, as well. So instead of feeling bad about the work I'm not getting done, I need to focus on everything I have accomplished.

To help with my attitude adjustment, I've committed to two things—a minimum of thirty minutes of exercise per day, and going to bed by 10:30. It's difficult to keep my emotions in check without exercise and rest.

I needed to see my OB-GYN yesterday for a post-hysterectomy checkup. It was exactly one year and one week ago that I was showing him the lump in my right breast. I anticipated being more emotional than I was when I actually saw him again. He was the one who told me on the phone that it was cancer, yet he was very professional and matter-of-fact. My other doctors are much more emotional, while he's more stoic. I wanted to thank him for saving my life—so many other doctors would have just said, "You're nursing; don't worry about this little lump," or even, "Come and see me when you're done nursing your baby." I wanted to thank him for being calm and choosing his words so carefully when he called with the news. But I chickened out because I knew telling him these things would reduce me to a puddle of tears.

Next Friday is Wade's birthday, and my cousin Kelsey is getting married. Vivian is a flower girl—she's a vision in her white dress. Jackson is the ring bearer; he's unbelievably cute in his tux. This weekend, I'll try to find a dress for me. I also need to decide if I'll keep the blonde hair for the wedding. Keeping in mind that many family photos will be taken and we'll look at those for years to come, I need to make a decision. Keeping it blonde is a statement of rebellion that says, "Screw you, cancer!" Going brunette again is a statement that I'm ready to be myself again and want this moment in time to be remembered as getting my life back. With brunette hair in the photos, future generations may look at the photo with no knowledge of my journey. The blonde hair might inspire questions: "Didn't Grandma Camille have brown hair?" I'm considering a compromise of having blonde hair for the rehearsal dinner and brunette for the wedding. We'll see what I decide.

I'm dreading tomorrow because it's the one-year anniversary of my diagnosis. But I'm looking forward to hosting my one-year-survivor ice cream social celebration. Vivian is having a difficult time wrapping her brain around having a party for cancer. I'm sure that tomorrow she'll just be happy to be running around with her friends and eating ice cream.

Ice Cream Social

Sunday, September 14, 2008, 10:07 p.m.

Nobody was more surprised than I was that I got through the day without crying. Lately, tears are coming so easily that I'm beginning to resemble Tammy Faye Bakker, complete with the black mascara tear tracks down my cheeks.

All day was highly scheduled, which helped. The morning started with returning to teaching Sunday school for the first time since my chemo-induced hiatus. The energy of those little preschoolers and kindergarteners is wonderful. My favorite moment was when, as we wrapped up our prayers of thanksgiving, one little guy announced, "I'm grateful for poopie diapers!" Stifling laughter, I clarified that sharing prayers should be limited to things we're really grateful for rather than jokes that will make our friends laugh. Thinking about it now, I'm guessing God got a good laugh out of that prayer too.

After church, the ice cream social was held in the church basement. A nice representation of people from my family, neighborhood, church, and work were there. It was perfect. After that, my mom joined us for errands and dinner. Then I went to the gym.

The past year has felt more like three years. It's included so much sadness, but more than that, I've learned that no matter what goes wrong in life, we're surrounded by people who really do want to help. That's a great comfort.

MRI Fiasco

Wednesday, September 17, 2008, 9:51 p.m.

I keep thinking this whole thing will start to get easier, or at least I'll somehow get used to it, but the opposite is true. Today was a difficult day. I went for a breast MRI at 7:30 this morning. An MRI once a year is included in routine surveillance for BRCA2-positive women.

The good part of working to live in the moment is that I don't really fret over these tests and doctors' appointments for days in advance anymore. However, once I changed into the hospital gown (and hospital pants too—what a treat!), my emotions surprised me. After the technician started the IV for the contrast dye, I started to cry. The tears were triggered by the memory of my last MRI. That's when they told me after the procedure that I could no longer nurse Jackson. Not even one more little "here's the last time, buddy" weaning. Last year, I cried all through the MRI, and this year I did, as well. I wonder if I'll always cry with this specific medical test.

Today, after I pulled myself together from being sad about last year's MRI, the tech positioned me on the machine. It's a precarious facedown position with your arms and legs held up by various vinyl-covered foam pieces. Some of these foam chunks were pressing on my ribs, making breathing awkward. Plus, after six weeks of being conditioned in radiation to not move or breathe while in the machine, I started to hold my breath. That's not sustainable for the forty minutes an MRI takes. Even before the first image, I pressed the call button in a panic. My recollection of the last MRI is that my head wasn't in the machine, so when my entire body including my head went into the machine, I felt totally claustrophobic. The tech offered oxygen, which I refused at first because I couldn't imagine a mask strapped to my face, as well. She brought over the oxygen, which luckily, was just a little tube that sat in the area under my face, so I could direct it however I wished. Once I pulled myself together, the test started. Although they give you headphones with music, once the machine starts up, the knocking and buzzing is so loud you can't hear a thing from the headphones. I felt shell-shocked as if I'd been in a war zone with all that knocking and buzzing. The entire experience was totally miserable. I felt as if I couldn't breathe—just thinking about it now puts me in a panic.

Tonight, we went to an impromptu barbecue for my cousin Kelsey, who's getting married on Friday. Just as we arrived, my plastic surgeon, Dr. Nicholson called. I forgot that I'd called him last week with some questions, but he was out of town. After asking Dr. Nicholson all my questions, we came to the bottom line—regardless of the method we select for reconstruction, all the various methods exist for aesthetic rather than medical reasons. In other words, I can choose whatever I wish without risking my health one way or another. This gave me no further clarity on the choice between lat flaps and tissue expanders, but at least I better understand the risks and benefits of both types of reconstruction. It's a choice between possible long-term complications for short-term comfort. I still need more time to make the decision. It could come down to flipping a coin.

Tomorrow night is Kelsey's rehearsal dinner, and the wedding is on Friday. I hope to wake up a little early tomorrow to practice Vivian's updo just one more time before the big day. Can't wait to see her and Jackson in their flower girl and ring bearer clothes!

Panic Attack

Friday, September 19, 2008, 4:55 a.m.

Ever since Wednesday's MRI fiasco, I've been riddled with anxiety. That night as I prepared for bed, I was overcome by a sensation of suffocation. Not just a feeling of trouble getting a good deep breath, but feeling like a fish out of water unable to breathe at all. Opening a bedroom window helped quite a bit, and finally I fell asleep.

Then Thursday morning while sitting at my desk at work, I had some type of panic attack. Again, I felt as if I couldn't breathe. The tears started flowing, and I wasn't sure what to do. Remembering the open window from the night before, I thought a breath of fresh air would help. The balcony door near my desk was locked for an event. It's five stories down to get outside the building, and I couldn't imagine walking so many steps. I wanted to call Wade, but what was he going to do from across town? Three of my coworkers were standing nearby, so I went up to them. Immediately, they saw I wasn't myself, and when I described what was happening, they were quick to talk me down off the figurative ledge, and most importantly, they made me laugh. Within a few minutes, I felt like myself again.

The experience of troubled breathing morphed into a weird type of claustrophobia by early evening. It was like I was trapped by my own skin, as if I might be suffocated by my skin. Everything felt too tight, including my shoes. As I dressed for the rehearsal dinner, I realized I couldn't possibly wear the dress I'd intended because it would add to the feeling of suffocation. Instead, I wore the most comfortable bra I own with an ugly loose dress and flat shoes. It was the only way to feel physically comfortable, but I had to sacrifice the social grace of wearing a cute dress and heels for this special occasion. It stinks to see everyone looking their best when I'm looking my worst. Thank goodness everyone is looking at the kids and not me.

Years ago, I heard that suicides increase in the springtime. While I don't know if this report was true, it said the reason is this: most people are happy and feeling renewed because winter is finally ending. But those with depression feel worse because they're not feeling renewed, instead having to watch everyone else transformed and happy. At the rehearsal dinner last night, I felt happy for Kelsey and her groom, Justin, and it's delightful to see Vivian out of her mind with excitement to be a flower girl. Yet it's hard for me to surrender to the joy of the occasion. My anxiety coats me with a social awkwardness. Plus, it's weird to relate on more than a surface level to anyone who isn't reading these "postcards from Camp Chemo" here on CaringBridge. By telling people on CaringBridge what's going on, I feel like then I can live in the moment when we're together in person—because all my cancer experiences are already out there.

Some people I'm very close to don't read these CaringBridge posts, which I can respect. My former self would've never been able stomach reading about all of this, and I'm continually amazed at the readers who stick with me. However, it's strange to show up with my compression bandage and have people wonder why my arm is wrapped up. My wrapped arm is ancient history to me, but to them, it's a new development that requires an explanation that I don't want to provide.

I used to be constantly bent on self-improvement. Now I'm just trying to make it through each day without emotionally crumbling.

Even looking at old photos of myself is painful. My long, dark hair has become a symbol of a person I used to be, but now it seems forever out of reach. I didn't know how great I looked at the time, and now I would give anything to turn back the clock.

In addition to feeling like so many of my positive qualities are slipping between my fingers, my hope for the future is also slipping away. I'm convinced this cancer will metastasize, and I'll be given a death sentence.

Rationally, I tell myself, this is a terrible way to live. Why am I wasting healthy days thinking these horrible thoughts? Sitting at the rehearsal dinner last night, I wondered if I'd live long enough to see Vivian or Jackson get married. While nobody has a guarantee of one more day on this earth, I have an extra set of ticking statistical time bombs. It's a vicious downward spiral—to love life, fear losing it, and then love it a little less each day but never stop fearing the loss of it. After all, this is the only life we know. It's unfortunate that my spiritual world, which might help me navigate this complex territory, has been like a desert, dry and lacking life-giving water.

The wedding today makes me pause and think how life has changed. At age seven, I was a flower girl for my cousin Sunny, and now at age seven, my own daughter is a flower girl for Sunny's daughter, Kelsey. I don't want my stress to ruin anything for Vivian, so just for today, I'll breathe deeply, forget my worries, exercise, and even though it may feel like it, I'll believe—just for today—that I won't suffocate in my own skin.

Suicidal Thoughts
Saturday, September 20, 2008, 11:30 p.m.

Something strange is happening to me. I've been thinking about suicide. How totally insane to think about killing myself because I'm afraid of getting a terminal diagnosis of metastatic breast cancer. I would never actually attempt suicide, but when I pass by a sharp object in the kitchen, I have this weird thought—or maybe it's better described as an impulse—like *What would happen if I put that in my neck?* I conclude that it would really hurt, and that's enough to stop me. Why on earth would I do anything that would require even more medical intervention? Haven't I already had enough?

I've also been feeling angry with the kids lately. I've been ready to smack them for doing nothing, but I would never actually do it. It's weird to even think about hitting them; I've never hit them and don't agree with it as a parenting strategy, so these impulses are foreign to me.

What was once a strong faith in God has vanished. Growing up, my mom took me to church every week, read Bible stories to me, and made sure I said prayers at night. That built a strong foundation of faith for me, and I'm so thankful to my mom for her commitment. But now it seems that foundation has crumbled. I have no idea how to restore my faith, or even if it's necessary. I wish that my feelings were more positive, like they were before the cancer.

Thankfully, none of Kelsey's wedding photos I've seen so far included me. I don't know why I insisted the photographer take a family picture of Wade, the kids, and me. Well, actually, I do. I was thinking that if something happens to me, then at least the kids will have some professional photos. My younger self would never believe how my waistline and life have turned out. So different from what I'd planned.

Feet in the Bed

Monday, September 22, 2008, 5:02 a.m.

Two hours 'til sunrise, and I'm wondering, how many feet can one bed hold? The king-sized bed was holding twelve feet before I got up. Here's our pattern—one of us will put Jack to sleep in our bed so the count begins with his two feet. Then Wade and I will go to sleep, adding our two pair. Around 4:00 a.m., Vivian stumbles into our bed, increasing the combined foot count to eight. A few hours later, Rocko joins us, purring violently, with his four little feet. Cedric, our white cat, soon joins the party and puts the foot count up to sixteen. Our pretty dog, Savannah, is banned from the bed, though. She's way too big to fit in with the sixteen feet already occupying the bed. Poor girl.

Lately, the kids have been fighting over who gets to snuggle Mommy. The other night when I was so sad, Wade pointed out that "everyone wants to lay hands on Mommy." It's sweet to think of all the times I've laid my hands on my little children to soothe their pain from scrapes, hurts, or restlessness. Now on some level, they want to return the favor. Our oldest cat, Dr. Rocko, also wants to get close to me—I think he senses my emotional pain. Regardless of how I'm feeling, though, this morning, my two feet needed to get out of that crowded bed. Once our upstairs remodel is finished and the children have their own bedrooms, we resolve to enforce a stricter "no kids in bed" policy that will leave us all more room to sleep.

We received word just yesterday that my MRI showed nothing unusual. A clean bill of health almost makes the nasty test worth it. While breath hasn't been coming easily to me in the last few days, including this morning, I'm able to relax and not panic so that I can focus on getting enough oxygen.

The past few days have been a time of diving down to explore the depths of all that worries and upsets me. It reminds me of all the times I left this world for a thin place during my chemo comas. The miracle is that I've been able to surface once again. I've rediscovered the thin line that keeps us all within the boundaries of this life, of beauty, and of love. The other day when I was feeling so troubled, I noticed a lawn sign that had two ballot-style boxes, with one word next to each box—hope and fear. The imaginary voter had already put a red check mark in the box next to hope. While clearly there was a political message to the sign, it rang true as a simple life philosophy: How many times in life must we choose between hope and fear? How many times have I made that choice in the past year? The depression and anxiety I feel at times are real. I know there's a brain chemistry component I can't choose, but eventually, I need to decide how long to stay in that murky place. The decision is about finding the help I need. That being said, Wade has really had my back the last few days. Instead of taking my antisocial behavior personally, he was quick to find several ways to reassure me. Yesterday, he dedicated the day to me, doing all the things I normally wish for on a Sunday. He went to church with me. Then our babysitter came to watch the kids while we took a long walk (almost two hours). Then we went clothes shopping for me. The walking—and the knowledge that I now have a bunch of new short-sleeved shirts that work with my massively bandaged arm—did much to improve my mood.

Wade and I also talked about the future. Sometimes I'm so certain that the cancer will return that the future seems impossible. But we made a decision to listen to my doctors, who say I have a good chance of making it to old age. We started imagining a series of vacations we'd like to take. We'd love to visit Paris, the South of France, and Italy. Another dream vacation is visiting a dude ranch out west. Dreams and plans for the future, like remodeling our house, are leaps of faith. The renovation represents a vote for hope over fear. It's the hope for a better tomorrow, and as Wade's dad, Gene, pointed out, it's a dream that can help us get through the MRIs and other upcoming medical hurdles. I also love that these are goals our family can dream together. It's a way to bring warmth and love to us all without having to share the same bed!

Anniversary
Wednesday, September 24, 2008, 9:19 p.m.

Today marked one year since my lumpectomy. Exactly one year ago, we got the news the cancer had spread to the lymph nodes. One year ago today, we learned I would need chemo and radiation. All these things were heavy to hold at the time, but a year later, it's actually more difficult because the cumulative effect has made the loss of innocence complete.

I saw my oncology psychologist this afternoon to tell her about my panic attacks. She explained many helpful things, but the bottom line is these anniversaries are causing some post-traumatic stress. She gave me many practical ways to cope—for example, telling myself, "I'm safe," if I start to have breathing trouble again. She also suggested I take the time for right-brain activities, such as exercise, writing, and savoring the moments with the kids. The panic attack is my brain saying, "Pay attention to this hurt," after I've been trying to ignore it for so long.

The other day as I sat down for lunch with a friend at a restaurant, a woman sitting next to us noticed my compression bandages and asked, "Do you have lymphedema?" She's the first person I've met who has actually known what is wrong with my arm. She showed me her own arm, which was very swollen. Her husband used to help with her bandaging, but after he died, she gave up on wrapping it. She asked if I did my own bandaging, and I told her yes. I also gave her the name of my lymphedema doctor. My lunch companion told me after we left that she'd overheard the woman say to her friend, "Maybe I'll visit that doctor. If she can do her bandaging, so can I." It made me feel good to know I'd had a positive impact on someone. It also made me feel a little scared to see someone with such a puffy arm. It is tempting to give up on all the bandages, exercise, and physical-therapy appointments, but now I'm even more determined to see it through.

Wade and I had an appointment yesterday with the breast surgeon, Dr. Ingamar, who works with my plastic surgeon, Dr. Nicholson. We finalized the decision to go with Dr. Nicholson and Dr. Ingamar. Dr. Farah doesn't work with Dr. Nicholson, and I'm sad to not have him care for me again, but I'm relieved that we've finally made the decision to schedule the mastectomy and reconstruction. It had been smoldering in the back of my mind for weeks, feeding my anxiety. Our plan is to enjoy the holidays and Vivian's birthday. Then we hope to schedule my final surgery for January 15. It's unlikely that the hospital, breast surgeon, and plastic surgeon's schedules will align for that exact date, but anytime close to that will work. Dr. Ingamar emphasized that three weeks of recovery is pushing it; six weeks is a more realistic expectation. When I told her that I bounce back really quickly, she informed me that this procedure is different; they'll be moving muscles around in my body, and I'll feel like I've been hit by a truck for quite some time.

Brunette Again

Sunday, October 5, 2008, 10:56 p.m.

At long last, I'm brunette again. The color itself is a disappointing reddish brown. It looks OK, but it's not the color I wanted. I wanted my rich, dark brown back. I'll try another box of color in a week or two. Wade has said so many times that he's glad to have me looking more like myself.

What I really sought in that box of hair color is my identity. Like a teenager experimenting with new looks to find a bridge from childhood to adulthood, I'm trying desperately to find the right identity to bridge life before cancer into life after cancer. If only it were just my hair that required retooling—but it's so much more than that. It's my career, my volunteer work, my family life, how I care for my body, how I spend every minute of my time, and how I spend every penny of my money. All these elements of my life need reexamination and reinvention. The process is exhausting. This struggle for identity is pressed against the backdrop of appalling urgency—I now understand that my time is short. While my prognosis is good and we have every reason to believe I'll live to age seventy, I can no longer take time for granted. I can't put off doing the things that will make the world better today. But I must balance this new reality with the day-to-day obligations of the life I built before cancer—and with the resources that have been stretched so thin during my illness.

One of my favorite writers is Flannery O'Connor, a genteel Southern woman who wrote with violent ferocity. I heard this quote from her years ago: "You shall know the truth, and it shall make you odd." I've discovered many truths during cancer treatment, and many of them probably do make me appear to be quite odd. That's something I need to claim as part of my new identity. Today, I'm unafraid to speak truth to others and to myself.

This week, I graduated from physical therapy—and received permission to ditch the bulky compression bandages, just in time for winter and long sleeves, which would have never fit over the bandages. Instead of bandages, I must wear my compression sleeve during the day, and I got a new bulky black sleeve to wear at night. Imagine a black oven mitt that extends all the way up to the shoulder. It's custom-made based on measurements of my arm. This nighttime sleeve even has my name sewn onto the tag. I'm told it should be covered by my insurance. I hope so, because it cost $900, which is way more than I paid for my wedding dress. Amazing. Perhaps they should sew some pearls and lace onto it to make it at least seem more worthy of a wedding-gown price tag.

Surgery Scheduled
Wednesday, October 15, 2008, 3:52 a.m.

So much has been happening lately. Another survivor recently pointed out how life has changed for us. When most people attend a funeral, they'll have a heightened awareness of the fragility of life. They may even make resolutions to improve their lives. Then after two or three days, work or kids or various tasks will pull them back to the way things were before, and they'll return to business as usual. Cancer survivors don't go back to life as usual after their brush with mortality.

A few days later, I had a follow-up conversation with this same survivor and asked, "Is living in this heightened awareness sustainable?" We both agree that it's not. The burden of feeling a sense of urgency to make each day count is overwhelming. This survivor also explained that during chemo or after a surgery, we can only do so much in a given day. The scant resources of energy and alertness limit our activity to the extent that these limits can provide an organizing principle. Now that my full energy is pretty much back, what's my new organizing principle? I have so much life to make up for, but I'm living in a new reality.

I need to make some choices. This same wise survivor advised me at the start of chemo to decide what's most important for me, because I can't do it all. I chose work and family. Everything else was put on hold. Now, once again, I need to prioritize. Work and family remain at the top of my list. Everything else will need to take a backseat until life moves into balance.

Yesterday, my mastectomy and reconstruction surgery was scheduled for January 15. In a weird way, I'd been looking forward to this for so long, but I felt very emotional as we finally set the date. The sense of dread for the six weeks of painful recovery feels overwhelming.

Last fall and winter, I looked forward to a better life once summer arrived. This fall and winter, again I'm looking forward to a better life once summer arrives—my surgery will be done, my expanders (which will be in for six months) will be out, and my implants will be in. So with any luck, I can run around in cute summer clothes, braless and carefree. That's one advantage of fake breasts—no bra is required because they remain forever perky on their own.

Looking ahead to the summer reminds me that the change from summer to fall has always been difficult for me. I don't have clinical seasonal affective disorder, but I do suffer from darker moods and less energy as the light declines every fall. This year, I'm really noticing my thinking change with the season change, and I can't tell if it's the season, menopause, PTSD, or cancer. Such lovely choices.

On Friday, when I should have been working, I was on the phone with my insurance company and a lymphedema compression sleeve company. After about an hour of going back and forth about insurance coding, I started to cry while talking to the woman at the compression sleeve company. I said maybe I should just pay the bill (it's only $115) and get my life back. She explained that I shouldn't pay it, because under federal law, I'm entitled to this. She's going to recode it and submit again. Hopefully, this time it will work. Everyone at my health insurance company has been great, but it gets so confusing—and I have a master's degree in communication, for heaven's sake. It really shouldn't be so difficult. I remembered a statistic about people filing bankruptcy—a big percentage of the filings are because of medical bills. My experience that day made me wonder how many of these expenses would have been covered by insurance. I can imagine how all the phone calls to insurance companies, along with doctors' appointments, plus working and family needs, could just make many people give up. I will forever respect people who live with chronic conditions and have to fight with insurance companies on a regular basis. At least I can imagine a time in my life when all of this will ease up.

Yesterday, a crew of guys ripped off the siding and roof of our house. The demo day was perfectly in line with how I'm feeling emotionally—like somehow my life is being deconstructed. The upside is that we'll have a house that's going to be much better suited for our family, including my mom, in the near future. Once the construction is complete, we'll have three bedrooms and a bathroom upstairs for the four of us, and then our existing two bedrooms and bathroom will be a perfect mother-in-law apartment so my mom can sell her house and move in. She'll have her own entrance, so she can feel like she has her own place. She's healthy, but she's ready to sell her house, and we're ready to have her closer. It takes twenty minutes for her to get between our houses, which doesn't seem like a lot, but she's here at least five days a week to help with the kids or with me. We'll be so happy to have her here. The single parent–only child bond I share with my mom is strong. My mom always wanted a son in addition to her only daughter. When I married Wade, she really felt she had gained that son. The two of them get along so well. I'm glad we'll be able to return some of the generosity she's shared with us.

At the office, work has been flowing beautifully. It's amazing how much I can accomplish without the constant interruptions of doctor and physical-therapy appointments.

A while back, I had planned to take a couple of half days off work for some personal time, but I needed to put that off until my doctor appointments slowed down. Now I look forward to being able to schedule a little time off here and there. I'll find out in a few days if I'll emerge from my surgical leave with any remaining vacation or if I'll need to use all my vacation days before my short-term disability can start. Thinking about taking healthy time off work is a fun diversion.

Today's Sermon

The pumpkins are carved, the cold wind is whipping at the windows, and our front-yard skeletons and ghosts are in position. It's once again the time of year when we, the living, remember those who have gone before and poke fun at our deepest fears. Tonight, the cold, spooky wind makes me feel so cozy inside our little house. I should say our little house that has grown so much. In the past two weeks, we've gained an entire second story to the house. Workmen have been coming over every morning. Thank goodness we hired our friend and neighbor Steve as our contractor—it could be unsettling to allow a stranger such full access to our house and our disorganized life.

Seeing the siding and roof pulled off our house felt like a good analogy for my upcoming mastectomy. Everything will be pulled apart and laid bare. Then, when all the potentially hazardous tissue has been removed, I'll be reconstructed into something better and (hopefully) bigger, just like our house has become bigger and better. Wade and Vivian really wanted the siding on the house to be red, but given my chemo-induced aversion to red, we decided on blue. My blue-averse grandmother wouldn't be pleased, but my mom assures me it's OK to select the color we want.

I've been struggling with depression again. During the workday, I can function, but when I'm with the kids, my fuse is shockingly short. Most often when I look into the future, I see my life in shambles—Wade has left me, and the cancer has returned. The dark thoughts and lack of patience make it hard to recognize myself. Sometimes it seems as if I'm watching someone else, and it's upsetting to feel so lost. Wade is wonderfully understanding. He's been clearing the way at home for me to have as much time to relax as possible. I'll see a new doctor, a psychiatrist, in two weeks. I have faith he'll find the right medications to get me back to myself again.

Today, our priest closed his sermon with an essay I recently wrote on charitable giving:

For some reason, I can't seem to get myself too worked up about this financial crisis. I understand that we're in a recession. I know people will lose their jobs. Others will postpone retirement. Finding work will become more difficult. It will take years for the economy to recover from this turmoil.

Yet despite the gloomy outlook and our shrinking 401(k) balances, I still feel like I have it pretty good. My husband and I are employed. My cancer is being held at bay with minimal treatment. If I need more medical intervention, it's available. When it comes to the big stuff, we're doing well.

Overall, we feel blessed. But we still have some anxiety. Our incomes fluctuate because we both work on commission. We don't have any financial cushion—we lack the three to six months of living expenses in savings that financial advisors recommend. Our first instinct to deal with this crisis is to increase our savings and slash our charitable giving, because it's a pretty easy item to delete from the spreadsheet. However, upon further examination, we've made the choice as a family to increase our charitable giving this holiday season.

Last Christmas season, I was undergoing chemotherapy for breast cancer, and my heart broke as I considered all the people in the world who need treatment and will never receive it. This Christmas season, we have the opportunity to donate money for a new medical clinic in Uganda through our church and the Minnesota nonprofit Give Us Wings. Last year, we were struggling to meet our out-of-pocket deductible. This year, we have the opportunity to participate in both the clinic and an adopt-a-family program to brighten the holidays for another family.

Even in this the poor economy, we're doing well. Many people will pull back on their gifts to charity this year. The need for charitable services will increase as the economy falters. This sounds like a recipe for disaster. We can do something about it, so we'll step up our giving. As long as we have jobs, we'll continue to give to worthy causes. If everyone who is doing OK will just lend a hand to those who need it, we'll all get through this crisis.

As the priest read, he got a little choked up during part of it. At the end, Wade whispered, "How do you feel, now that you've made the priest cry?" After the service, several people said my essay inspired them. How strange to be buoyed by my own words: yes, we can make it through this economic crisis, and I can make it through this difficult time.

I've been so tired, sleeping nine to ten hours per night. The change of seasons has always done a number on me, this year more than ever. On Thursday, I'll see my oncologist for my quarterly check-in. He'll look at my blood levels to make sure nothing is amiss. The other day, I heard that a friend of a friend, someone much younger than I am, got bad news at her quarterly checkup—her cancer has metastasized. While I know it does no good to worry, it's hard not to.

The house construction and Halloween will be welcome distractions this week.

Joining the Club
Tuesday, October 28, 2008, 4:52 a.m.

Today, I'll see my oncology psychologist. Already, I've come such a long way since the panic attacks in the MRI machine. Hope is mostly eluding me these days. However, considering how far I've come since that day, I can be hopeful about getting back to myself within a few more weeks. It's difficult to articulate how lonely I feel—and, like cancer, depression is something people find difficult to discuss. Inquiring about an acquaintance's broken arm or cold is easy, but asking about someone's cancer or depression means you risk hearing a much longer story than you'd bargained for—and we don't know how to help the afflicted. Now that I've become so experienced with both cancer and depression, I still don't always know what to say.

Just yesterday, I was left speechless when a woman I admire called to say she'd "joined my club." All I could say was, "Oh geez, that really sucks. I'm so sorry to hear that." I went to see her, and it was like walking into my past. There she sat with a sheet of notes from her doctor's phone call, confusion, and innocence swirling around all the questions that won't be answered for weeks. I gave her a list of my favorite doctors, nurses, and hospitals. One of the first things I told her is that she'll be amazed by the community that will surround her family to lift them up. We discussed genetic testing, staging, and surgery.

What I didn't tell her is that the journey is long. The struggles continue even after the long process of surgery, chemo, and radiation has ended. The body is ravaged by the side effects of medication and procedures. Then with each treatment for the side effects come more side effects. I didn't want to tell her that there may be times when she won't know herself or that sometimes she may feel worthless. Depression is a reality for many dealing with cancer. Death lingers, waiting around the corner.

This newly diagnosed family's innocence was apparent in their confusion over what to make of the diagnosis. It reminded me of the innocence our family had as we embarked on this journey. While it's sad to lose innocence, it's replaced by experience. Would I trade the experience I've gained for the innocence I once had? Today, yes, I would. At other times, I wouldn't, because I cherish the lessons I've learned along the way. So strange that this hypothetical question is even asked by cancer survivors—would I go back to life before cancer? Would I trade it in? They're not logical questions, because the choice isn't real. It isn't our decision to make. Yet by asking the question, we're forced to examine our lives and discover the good that has come along with the bad.

My prayer life has been very strained. I have someone new to pray for now, and suddenly, prayer came easily, and that provides a sweet relief.

Fashion Faux Pas

Sunday, November 2, 2008, 3:21 a.m.

When I was pregnant with Vivian, I wanted to learn all I could before she was born so nursing would go well. I read *The Womanly Art of Breastfeeding*. At the time, a four-hundred-page book about a totally natural process seemed crazy. But when Vivian arrived, and the complicated nature of nursing became apparent, that book was a godsend. Recently, a friend loaned me a four-hundred-page volume about menopause, and I thought, *Why do I need four hundred pages about hot flashes?* Now that I'm in the thick of menopause, though, I'm referring to that book with renewed interest.

My psychologist suggested that my emotional struggles are in large part hormonal. As estrogen leaves the body during menopause, the natural desire to nurture fades. From a biological standpoint, the body has completed reproduction and is preparing to die. It turns out my desire to leave a legacy, to focus on work and myself, is more normal than I'd thought. This is a typical stage women go through during menopause. Most go through menopause when their children are grown, so it's OK to focus on one's legacy, but with two small kids, I need to keep my focus on raising them. Good thing they have such a capable dad and a caring grandma, so when my nurturing eludes me, Wade and my mom can nurture the kids. As for understanding that some of my emotional issues are hormonal, sometimes just knowing why something is happening makes it easier to navigate.

The meeting with my oncologist didn't help my emotional issues so much. He seemed distracted and stressed—and I can't blame him. Oncology must be the most stressful of the medical specialties. Still, the experience left me cold when I wanted to be reassured. I want him to heal my quality of life, but that's not in his job description. I know he cares about me as a person, but he isn't trained like the psychologist, nor does he have the time to attend to my complicated emotional states. As long as I'm still breathing, he's done his job. The next day, he called to say my blood levels are good—no signs of cancer. My thyroid and vitamin D levels aren't in such good shape, both of which could be contributing to my darker mood. Increased thyroid medication and vitamin D supplements should help.

It felt like Christmas yesterday when my new lymphedema compression sleeves arrived in the mail. The ones I got in July went in the garbage. The insurance finally agreed to pay for the new sleeves after my diligent phone calls. The key was finding a new supplier willing to code the transaction in the way the insurance company wants. It was a hassle to make all those phone calls, but I'm happy to have "cracked the code" so now I can have what I need at least until the end of this year. Who knows what will change after the first of the year. The rules change every year, just to keep us sickos on our toes.

Part of caring for my lymphedema is making sure the skin on my right arm and hand stays clean and intact. I've noticed the skin on my hand has already started to get very dry and is showing surface cracks. Any break in the skin could lead to another flare-up, more bandages, and physical therapy. Worst-case scenario, it could land me in the hospital with a terrible infection. I'm highly motivated to keep my skin in good shape, but already it looks like it will be a challenge.

There are so many things in my closet that weren't there a year ago, some due to these lovely compression garments. Despite all these new items, I'm still a walking fashion faux pas. It makes me realize how this illness has permeated all aspects of my life. The sports bras and camisoles during radiation when a regular bra was too hard on my burned skin. The short-sleeved tops because long sleeves wouldn't fit over my compression bandages. The clothes, a size bigger thanks to the chemo weight gain. The lightweight layers to deal with menopause-induced hot flashes. Only my most comfortable shoes work these days, because my big toenails are in danger of falling off from the chemo. Who knew this process would change my fashion sensibility so much? My transformed closet is a good metaphor for all the changes that have happened in the past year.

"Gone Self"

Thursday, November 6, 2008, 6:24 p.m.

Before cancer, I had thyroid problems. For many years, I've been treated by Dr. Park, an endocrinologist. My thyroid concerns were put on the back burner while addressing the cancer, but now it's time for me to address any thyroid issues that could be adding to my symptoms of depression.

I went into the endocrinology clinic expecting to see Dr. Park, but instead, his partner, Dr. William, was scheduled to meet with me. They didn't have any health records since my last visit over a year ago, so she took down my recent history—namely, the lumpectomy, chemo, and radiation. I hated rehashing my cancer history. As we started talking about my current thyroid issue, I blurted out, "Oh, and I had a hysterectomy in June." Funny that I'd totally forgotten to tell Dr. William about the hysterectomy as she updated my history.

I was there to give them the paperwork on my thyroid levels from the oncology clinic and to find out if my existing prescription is still relevant. Instead, she reminded me of other blood levels that my oncologist hadn't ordered. She couldn't give me what I came for—I need more labs first. Great. Another blood draw.

At my last visit with Dr. Park, the purpose of which was to check my thyroid levels, I also asked for some diet pills. Back then, at 131 pounds, I wasn't happy with my weight. I wanted to lose ten pounds for my high school reunion—ha, I'd celebrate 131 pounds now! Today, when Dr. William left the exam room, Dr. Park came in. He hugged me and asked, "How are you?" I started to sob.

Everything I've learned, all the writing I've done, every measure of love I've received in the last year, I would trade it to be that woman in a doctor's office complaining about wanting to lose ten pounds before her high school reunion. I might even sell my soul to go back. It's completely insane to consider returning to my old life. I know it's impossible, yet I continue to long for it. Somehow, I need to mourn the loss of my "gone self." This is what makes cancer survivors so desperate for a cure—it's maddening to consider anyone else having to go through this ordeal.

I cried all the way to work after seeing Dr. Park. I just couldn't stop. Once again, it was one of my wise, caring colleagues who threw down a rope and pulled me out of my pit of despair. And again, work provided a distraction that kept me calm for the rest of the day.

I accept that I'm mourning the loss of my life without cancer—that precancer perspective, that precancer woman. But today, I'm something new. I get to create my new life. What I create needs to be spectacular, so if I ever meet my "gone self" face-to-face, I can reassure her: your best is yet to come.

Great Escapes
Sunday, November 9, 2008, 4:47 p.m.

Friday night, I had the opportunity to visit a friend in the hospital. It's the first time I've visited someone else in the hospital since all my own hospital visits. I must admit, I was very happy to be the one doing the visiting, because after a few hours, I got to leave. That's the hard part of being the patient—you don't get to leave. This may seem obvious, but I've grown so accustomed to viewing everything from the patient perspective, I forgot how much easier it is to be a civilian.

A few days after visiting my friend in the hospital, I had my first psychiatrist visit, which was different from what I'd expected. Many of his questions were about physical symptoms, like sleep. This surprised me; I'd assumed he'd ask only questions about my mood. He'd like to prescribe a new antidepressant but needs to research and find one that won't cancel out my tamoxifen. He did write a prescription for Ativan, the antianxiety that helped me sleep during chemo. He suggested one pill in the morning and two before bed. I was really worried about taking it in the morning, because I associate it with going to sleep. But I took it yesterday morning, and I felt fine. It helped me keep my thoughts steady rather than drifting into uncomfortable territory.

He confirmed what I feel by saying he thinks it's silly when people say cancer is the best thing that ever happened to them. He acknowledged that regardless of how much I gain through the experience, life is just plain better without cancer. It was a relief to have him acknowledge this truth I've long suspected.

He confirmed that I've experienced textbook panic attacks and gave me some tips in case they happen again. He also explained that thoughts of suicide are not surprising within this context. It's not so much about wanting to die but rather a desire to escape. That rang true with me.

Without consciously realizing it, I've been wanting to escape. I've yet to run away to the Loews Miami Beach.

I was lucky to find two great escapes this weekend. The first was a fitness class that happened to be starting just as I arrived at the gym yesterday. It was very moderate exercise, and I only had to modify a couple of moves to prevent aggravating my lymphedema. I've been wanting to go to some classes—my former self enjoyed spinning and kickboxing classes—but those are out of the question until the lymphedema in my arm settles down.

Vivian designed the other great escape. She has no interest in restarting her music lessons that we had to quit during my treatment, but she's been asking for a sewing class for years. Finally, I found a good teacher, and we went to our first sewing lesson today. It is a beautiful studio in an old Victorian home. We made little drawstring bags appropriate for keeping jewelry or little stones. It was a very meditative experience to completely leave everything behind for two hours. The same with the exercise class—they were both times when I could shut off all other thoughts and escape into something beautiful and positive.

Snap Out of It
Monday, November 10, 2008, 9:56 p.m.

This ongoing struggle with poor mood continues to surprise me. I keep thinking I'll just snap out of it, but that isn't happening. The continued attention I must give my mental health is necessary, yet compared with physical symptoms, it would be easy to delay care. I suspect that ignoring my mental health contributed to my panic attack in the MRI machine. Now I'm on a varied regimen of increased exercise, new medication, right-brain activity, and relaxation, all designed to improve my mood. Feeling depressed much of the time is no way to live. While I acknowledge there's a chemical component over which I have little control, I'm determined to seize whatever control I can.

I've started again noticing beauty around me—the crisp, clean, cold air, the smell of burning wood that signals winter, the clementines in the grocery store, and Jackson coming at me at a full run to greet me with a hug at the end of the day.

I have hope that the scales will soon tip back to the side of feeling happy most of the time once again. But I must stay disciplined in my gratitude practice. At times, gratitude is the best solution for me. That and comedy. Which reminds me, it's time to watch *The Daily Show* for a good laugh at the world.

Nervous Breakdown

Friday, November 14, 2008, 8:04 p.m.

We're just barely hanging in there with my depression and the home re-model (we have a bathtub in the dining room at the moment, *très* white-trash chic)—and we're both very busy at work. A couple of days ago, I was thinking that if just one more thing is added to the load, everything will come crashing down. Then on Wednesday night, Vivian got sick. Throw-ing-up, high-fever sick. Fortunately, my mom was able to stay home with her on Thursday, and Vivian was well enough for school today. And the world didn't come crashing down.

Wade's level of selflessness continues to grow. It's as if he notices every little weight that falls upon my shoulders and tries to remove it. Tonight, he made a point of sitting down to watch a movie with the kids so I could have a little space to think.

The Ativan, vitamin D, increased exercise, and conscious positive thoughts have all been helping me improve my mood. Wednesday is my weekly dose of vitamin D. Wade thinks my mood improves for a few days after taking it.

During a conversation with a cousin, I learned that two paternal rel-atives suffered from a "nervous breakdown," as it was labeled back in the day. One was a successful merchant, new to America, whose busi-ness dried up during the Great Depression. He couldn't find work, and the only way they survived was thanks to money people owed them. He couldn't eat or sleep. When he was sent to the Mayo Clinic for help, they told him to go outside and walk three miles each day. He recovered and went on to live a successful life. Back in those days, the medications we now take for granted weren't available. I just can't imagine how I would have fared in those days. I guess it isn't worth pondering because I'd be dead already without modern-day cancer treatments.

I recently attended training at the museum to help with an arts program at Vivian's school. I signed up for the program last year, just before my diagnosis, and then had to bow out when we learned I'd need chemo. Now this year, I can participate in most of the program, but I won't be able to attend the class field trip to the museum because I'll be recovering from my mastectomy. So arriving at the museum training was bittersweet. I'm finally able to participate in the program, but I'm disappointed about missing the field trip and about having to skip the whole program last year. During the training, I recognized another participant as a woman who went to my high school. From across the room, she looked almost exactly the same as the last time I saw her more than twenty years ago. Before cancer, people used to tell me I looked exactly the same as when I was in high school. I felt so wistful that the same can't be said today. She still had her long, dark hair, though. She isn't someone I knew by name, only a familiar face, so there was no reason to say hello. Instead, I sat and imagined how easy her life must be, how lucky she is to still have her lovely long hair. It's dangerous business comparing how I feel on the inside to someone else's outsides. For all I know, she's a three-year cancer survivor, and her hair has grown back. Every moment I spend in self-pity is a wasted moment of my life, yet the temptation to feel sorry for myself increases. Maybe as I look back and realize the worst is behind me, it's finally safe to examine just how much has been lost. An old friend who is a soldier recently read this blog and said he now understands why cancer is called a battle. Just as I can't imagine the horrors of war, it's difficult to describe the full experience of cancer.

My darling little Jackson just crawled up in my lap and is driving his Matchbox car along the keyboard, so I guess now would be a good time to sign off. But first I have to brag about my other darling child. Vivian was the number-one seller in her school fund-raiser! I'm so proud of her and happy that despite all the disruptions in the past year, she can still excel.

Mozart

Sunday, November 16, 2008, 1:30 p.m.

Last night, I was reading some stories about coming close to death and healthy people interacting with people who are dying. The book, *Kitchen Table Wisdom* by Dr. Rachel Naomi Remen, is a series of short essays. Many of the stories reminded me of the thin places I experienced during chemo. While sometimes frightening and sad, when I was in a thin place, I felt closer to the divine than ever before. An overall sense of peace and well-being surrounded me. The prayers people said for me were palpable. I felt lifted on a wave of love. Despite experiencing horrible physical side effects, I rode on a wave of caring that made the suffering bearable. Now that the immediate physical danger is past and the worst of the side effects have diminished, I'm expecting myself to function as "normal." At times, I've even revved up to an accelerated pace, which isn't sustainable.

Reading Dr. Remen's essays last night made me realize that I'm longing for the spiritual connection that was so strong during the worst of my physical suffering. During chemo, I felt confident in my body's ability to heal; during radiation, God was just a prayer away. Now all things spiritual remain elusive. I reach out and find nothing.

However, after having deep spiritual experiences and coming so close to the divine, I'm left feeling like a drug addict searching for a fix. Can I fake it 'til I make it? Can I pretend to be cheerful and hopeful until I really feel those things again?

Before cancer, my fears centered around external threats—a stranger in a dark parking ramp, a society gone to anarchy, but now I fear that which is within me—not only stray cancer cells but the darkness of my own thoughts, my capacity for hopelessness.

This morning in church, the choir sang "Lux Aeterna" (Light Eternal) from Mozart's *Requiem*. The music is stirring, the words profound: "Let eternal light shine on us, Lord, as with your saints in eternity, because you are merciful. Grant us rest, Lord, because you are merciful." I believe some artists' hands are guided by God, and I believe Mozart was among them. He gives us a glimpse into heaven through pure beauty. As I listened to the music and words, I remembered that death is not an ending. I realized sadness and grief are just one part of saying good-bye to my gone self. It was only during the worst of my physical suffering that I was able to visit those thin places, feeling the hand of God gently, mercifully holding me. Now as I suffer in mind and spirit, I'm reminded that same merciful God is still holding me, his little child, in a warm embrace, saying, "It's OK. You're safe. I wish happiness and joy for you, my child." This most recent Mozart experience makes me so thankful that my mom instilled in me a love of both God and classical music. Her caring touch also helps me to remember my faith even when it feels far away.

I need to find an intentional practice to keep a remembrance of God close to my heart. I don't know what it will be, but I know I'll find it.

Dog Is My Copilot
Thursday, November 20, 2008, 8:41 p.m.

I've been getting cold. It's wonderful to get really chilled once again. Could menopause be loosening its wretched grip? I still have a hot flash a few times per week, but it's nothing like before. While I enjoy feeling cold when I'm indoors, the gray, cold outdoors is a drag.

Yesterday was D day—my weekly prescription dose of vitamin D. Placebo or no, my mood improves so much after taking it. In the hours I wasn't at work on Monday and Tuesday, I was crying. I even spent a little time crying at work. I took half a vacation day Tuesday and a half day today because Wade insisted I attend to my mental health. Turns out some time off and vitamin D are just what the doctor ordered. Today, I've gone through the entire day without a single despairing thought. I haven't wanted to throttle either child. The dog didn't annoy me today—in fact, I took her with me in the car when I picked up Jackson from school. I mostly like having the dog ride in my passenger seat because a) she looks really cute, and b) that "Dog is my copilot" bumper-sticker sentiment cracks me up. I laugh to myself each time I look over at her in the passenger seat.

Don't get me wrong; I'm not confident in my momentarily stable mind-set, but it gives me hope that I'll have a few good days. Unfortunately, each time I spiral downward, I seem to go further down.

On Tuesday, I saw a "healing coach." I'd made the appointment over a month ago when I was gung ho to lose weight, eat better, and improve my life by taking charge of my health. Instead of taking charge of anything, I cried the whole time I was in her office. I cried because I'd been feeling so proactive when I made the appointment, so ready for self-improvement—but today, there I was crying in her office because I'm hanging on by a thread—I can't even think about improving myself; I just need to get through the workday without crying.

She told me that I'm doing all that I can for my health right now, and the most important thing is to stabilize. "Be gentle with yourself; don't harass yourself because you can't do it all right now." Here I had fully expected her to sign me up for tai chi or convince me acupuncture is the way to better health. Instead, she suggested I increase visits to my psychologist and call the psychiatrist to nail him down for a new depression prescription. She also sent me home with a relaxation CD. I was sure the CD would annoy me. This CD is actually pretty good, though. It includes a walking meditation, which I tried on Tuesday evening in the halls of the high school where Vivian does her gymnastics class. I've listened to a couple of the guided imagery tracks and have felt much calmer afterward.

I'm looking forward to Thanksgiving next week. We'll relax in Iowa in a way we just can't relax at home. Especially these days with our home in such remodeling disarray—dust everywhere, junk everywhere. The walls have holes, and there's still a bathtub in our dining room. Oh, and dozens of boxes of bamboo flooring stacked up in our living room.

I have a suddenly wide-awake toddler at my side. Time to lie down with him and my relaxation CD, and drift off to my happy place . . .

Update
Saturday, December 13, 2008, 4:46 p.m.

Wade asked today if I've quit writing. It has been such a long time. A few weeks ago, I saw the psychiatrist again. It may seem ironic, but seeing the psychiatrist makes me feel less crazy. He gave me a prescription for a new antidepressant that I started taking two weeks ago. It's been working great—with no side effects! I love being able to cope with everyday life once again. I haven't cried for two weeks except for during a baptism at church. Baptisms always get me.

In addition to taking the antidepressants, I realized a few things about sadness. It's like the expression "You have nothing to fear but fear itself." When I was resisting the sadness and running away from it, like a shadow, it followed me just as quickly as I could run. But when I finally turned around, looked at it, and said, "You know, you have every right to be here. There is plenty to be sad about; I'm not going to deny you anymore," I was able to understand that sadness has a rightful place in my life now. Paradoxically, befriending the sadness has allowed it to take a backseat, and I've been able to resume my life.

In one month, I'll have my mastectomy. At work, I've been really moving fast so I can prepare for my recovery time. I've already achieved the most critical goals I set for myself to have done before my medical leave. There are still plenty of loose ends to tie up, but I'm relieved to have the most important things done. I'm also preparing internally. It's hard to explain, but I'm starting to focus inward a little bit more. Maybe feeling less chatty, more introverted. There is so much to process these days.

The main reason I haven't written is because we're going full speed to finish the house remodel. Or rather, Wade is going full speed; I'm just trying hard to keep up with the laundry and dishes and make sure the kids are out of his hair so he can work several hours each night and all day on the weekends. We only have until the second week in January to complete everything (as part of the mortgage deal), so we're spending every moment preparing for the holidays or working on the house.

A few weeks ago, I went to the holiday cabaret my company does each year. It's always an amazing performance. Most people play music or sing. I read a short, cleaned-up CaringBridge post. It was so enjoyable to get up and read for a live audience. I had to go really far back in the posts to find something that was even a little bit funny. Reading over what I've written really highlights how much more serious and depressing this journey has become over the last few months.

Another holiday party tonight, and more to come next weekend. It's nice to be present for all these parties, having missed them all last year.

Christmas Traditions
Wednesday, December 24, 2008, 2:29 p.m.

On this Christmas Eve, I'd like to share a little about our holiday traditions. We go to church with my mom at four o'clock. Then we all go to the big Christmas Eve party hosted by my cousin Melissa and her husband, Uri, where we eat like royalty and the kids open gifts. My other cousins Sunny her husband Mike, my cousin and godfather Mike, and his wife Ruth are usually there too. Some of my cousins' grown kids—Talia, Alexa, Kelsey, and Alec—attend when they're in town. Here's our other Christmas tradition: at some point in the evening, one of our kids will barf on Wade. Really. We have the ruined neckties to prove it. Last year, it was Jackson. The previous two years, Vivian did the honors. My money is on Vivian this year. She wasn't feeling well yesterday.

Christmas Day tends to be puke-free. It's generally a quiet day at our house with our little family and my mom. Gifts from Santa and Grandpa Gene and Grandma Beckie from Iowa are opened. We make a big breakfast and play with gifts all day.

As I gear up for next month's mastectomy, I have a happy update. Rewind to last week. A friend introduced me to her friend who'd had a mastectomy and reconstruction. We all had lunch together. This woman's story is similar to mine—she'd had radiation on one side, so the reconstruction was complicated. I told her my plans for a lat flap. She explained her reasoning for keeping her lat muscle whole by using a product called AlloDerm. My doctor mentioned it to me, and at a breast cancer conference a few months ago, one of the surgeons on the plastic-surgery panel said she used the product with most of her reconstructions. The surgeons describe AlloDerm as skin from a cadaver, which is sterilized and altered by removing cells and DNA to make it a simple tissue matrix that can be used in lieu of harvested muscle, keeping the patient's back muscles whole.

I asked the woman who'd chosen AlloDerm if she had to get past the idea of having skin from a cadaver used for her reconstruction. She said that the person who donated the skin wanted it to be used so someone else can live a better life. She feels like the donor is living on in her. Wow. I'd been thinking *cadaver*—death, decay, yuck. Now I'm thinking *donor*—generosity, legacy, beauty.

Two days later, I asked my plastic surgeon to tell me more about AlloDerm. Turns out, I'm a candidate to use it. Wade and I together decided it's the procedure we want. So instead of the lat flaps, I'll have AlloDerm and expanders that will eventually be replaced by implants. I'll be on the surgeon's table one hour less, in the hospital one day less, and should be back to work two weeks earlier. Plus, I won't have to rehab my back at all. The only possible downside is that if my body rejects the AlloDerm, we may have to go back and do a lat flap—which would mean an additional three to six weeks off work. However, my surgeon has never had to do that, so I'm confident about a good result. The only other downside is that I can't go any bigger than my existing cup size. I'd been planning to enhance my figure just a little bit. But we agree that a slightly smaller bustline is worth it in return for a lower risk of complications.

As we prepare to exchange Christmas gifts, I can report that I'm actually looking forward to my mastectomy, which will prevent new breast cancers. Plus, I'll receive a gift from a wonderfully generous person I'll never know.

New Year's Resolutions

Thursday, January 1, 2009, 9:50 p.m.

My mom asked if I've made any New Year's resolutions. "No way!" was my reply. Not this year. I've engaged in enough self-improvement this year to last a lifetime. Most years, I enjoy taking time to reflect on the past year and then contemplating how I can improve my life in the upcoming year. Now I just take each day as it comes.

Only two weeks until my mastectomy. My healing coach is sending someone from the in-patient integrative health team to stop by as they prep me for surgery. She'll work her voodoo to help me relax. Then she'll come back and see me after the surgery. I wonder if I'll wake up in a mass recovery room like I did with my lumpectomy. That was such a trip. The room was filled with beds of other recovering patients, I had an oxygen mask on my face, and I kept trying to remove it and get up. I kept thinking, *I need to escape.*

The nurse kept saying, "You need to keep that on," and "You need to stay here," as if I were a two-year-old, which was probably my mind-set at the time. I kept asking for my mom and dad, never mind that my dad died when I was young. Plus, I never called him Dad; I always used his first name. My mom raised me totally on her own. It was so weird to ask for my mom and dad!

As I prepare for a few weeks of low energy and reduced activity, I'm thinking of good reading material to have around—a book or two, a few magazines, and some sudoku and crossword puzzles. TV, radio, telephone calls, and visitors generally don't interest me when I'm recovering. I wonder if this time will be the same.

It's likely that I'll recover in our current bedroom even though the upstairs is almost ready. Wade continues to wow everyone with his carpentry skills. Our contractor is so impressed he's asked Wade to do some work with him. I'm not surprised—Wade works so hard, and he's so smart. It's amazing how he can look at something and then figure out how to make it. He would have been perfect in the pioneer days, when people had to make everything instead of buying things.

Tonight, I have an upset stomach from a new medication. Without giving too much information, let's just say I thought that any "female problems" would cease when my "female parts" were removed. On the contrary, when estrogen leaves the female body, the body revolts and becomes at times—well, rather revolting. The many secret joys of menopause.

Christmas was lovely and relaxing. Jackson squealed with joy as he opened his gifts. That's a memory I'll treasure forever. Vivian was so excited about New Year's Eve. We invited another family with two daughters to join us. We've been meaning to invite them over for a year, and the conversation was as enjoyable as we'd anticipated.

Today, we spent a lovely afternoon at my cousin Melissa's house. Lately, life has been somehow meeting my expectations. Without intentionally resolving to do so, I've started living in the moment once again. My happiness today doesn't depend on anything that's meant to happen tomorrow. Oh, and Wade got his Christmas Eve wish—a puke-free evening!

I'm the Healthy One Now

Monday, January 12, 2009, 9:23 p.m.

Right now, I'm really stressed out. In addition to my mastectomy on Thursday, Mike, my cousin Sunny's husband, had surgery on December 29, January 7, and then again today. Sunny was admitted to the hospital today with pneumonia, and she's on a ventilator and dialysis right now. Still another family member recently had a battery of medical tests. It's getting to be a bit too much. Just as I'm gearing up for my mastectomy, so many others in my family are falling ill. And these are people in the prime of life and otherwise healthy. It's very weird.

Against that sad backdrop, our home expansion happily passed the final inspection, so we complete the paperwork for the mortgage tomorrow. We have loads of touch-up work ahead, and it will take a while to move everything upstairs, but the project is complete in the eyes of the bank.

Vivian turned eight over the weekend, with eight screaming little girls helping her celebrate with a party. We played Bingo and Pass the Parcel, where each time the music stops someone unwraps one layer of paper on a gift. The person who unwraps the final layer wins the gift. Very exciting. Lots of screaming.

Tonight, I went with the kids to an Angel Foundation winter party. We had dinner, won prizes, the kids had their faces painted, and they decorated cookies with way too much frosting. Wade went to the hospital to be with my relatives. I went to the Angel Foundation party instead because I'm afraid that visiting a hospital could make me sick, which would mean postponing my mastectomy.

Sunny fell ill so suddenly, which is very disconcerting. It seems incomprehensible that someone could be healthy one day and then critically ill in the intensive care unit the next day. I keep thinking, *This is wrong. I'm the one who should be sick.*

I'd been feeling so good that I'd slowed down on the amount of anti-anxiety drugs I'd been taking. Earlier today, I realized I'm feeling anxious and should increase the dosage once again.

Sorry to be such a downer right now, but worrying about people you care about sucks. But then, I guess you already know how that feels. Thanks for caring about me.

Tomorrow

Wednesday, January 14, 2009, 9:24 p.m.

Last night, we slept upstairs in our new bedrooms. It was great!

That happy moment is tempered by Sunny's illness. Still kind of hard to believe that Sunny is so sick. Some relatives are coming in from out of town to visit her.

Jackson joined the illness club yesterday when he woke up with a sore ear and was diagnosed with his first-ever ear infection. Not bad to make it to age two and a half without an ear infection. The antibiotics are working their magic, and today he feels much better.

Tomorrow is the big day. Wade and I will leave for the hospital at 5:15 a.m. I've already said good-bye for a day or two to Vivian and my mom. Will give Jackson a kiss in the morning. I'm so glad my mom is always able to help with the kids. Her calming presence is a gift.

Thank you for all your well wishes and prayers. Please keep up the prayers. I'll be in the hospital for at least two nights and on heavy narcotics for at least one week. The drains that will be inserted in my chest under the skin will be removed after one to three weeks. From there, I think it's just a matter of incision care, pain management, and getting my energy back. That's the "no complications" scenario, which is what I'm banking on.

Overall, I feel pretty calm and just ready to go. The biggest concern is waking up on time to get to the hospital! Good thing Wade is an early bird.

A Happy and Sad Update

Monday, January 19, 2009, 10:13 a.m.

Hi, everyone, this is Wade writing for Camille today.

So sorry for the delay. The mastectomy and reconstruction went well, and the recovery is also going well. Camille is home but in a fair amount of pain, so she's sleeping most of the time. We received the best news we could have gotten—there was no cancer in any of the tissue that was removed.

Whew!!! Thank God!

Also good: there's no sign of infection. The hard work now is to get her out of pain and moving around a little bit more each day. Tomorrow will be her first outing—to the hairdresser to get a shampoo and maybe a cut if she can sit up that long.

Unfortunately, as she was recovering after the surgery on Thursday, Camille's cousin Sunny, who had gone into the hospital with pneumonia last week, passed away. This is awful for the entire family. Sunny was always the sweetest, most selfless person we knew. She is missed. Camille is having a hard time with this loss because the pain meds aren't allowing her to feel the emotions she thinks she should be and no doubt wants to be feeling. Also, she's missing the "remembrances" and get-togethers the rest of her family are having now. At least she's resting, right?

I feel like I should have a poignant quote or affirmation to insert here. I'm sorry, but I don't.

I wanted to also say thanks to my mom, Beckie, for coming all the way from Iowa to help so much with the kids and the laundry and the dishes and the food and the sweeping and the vacuuming. It was great to have you around for the support.

January of Misery
Thursday, January 29, 2009, 4:39 p.m.

As the anesthesia took effect two weeks ago today, Wade reports that while I drifted off, I asked for a kiss. After he gave me one, the nurses laughed as I said, "Oh, I like that! I want more kisses, honey." I was so happy that morning of the surgery—relieved that the day had finally come. The hospital nurses were commenting to me on how "perky" and happy I was acting before the surgery. That morning, I came up with a working title for my memoir, *Forever Perky*, which has a nice double meaning.

When I awoke in the recovery room, I was—again—so happy to realize I survived the surgery! I'm alive! That's how it is after surgery. I greet every doctor, nurse, and visitor with big smiles and warm words. But once the anesthesia starts to wear off, the pain and itchy skin starts, and it's more difficult to be cheerful.

The night of my surgery, my beloved cousin Sunny died. Mercifully, Wade and my mom waited until the next night to tell me the news. To understand this loss, it's important to know that I grew up with only my mom. No brothers and sisters. Just Grandma and Grandpa, my aunt Illeane, and her husband, my uncle Frank. Their four kids, Nina, Mike, Sunny, and Melissa were young adults when I was born, but they've always been so kind and treated me more like a younger sibling than a distant relative. Sunny was my favorite cousin. I spent my childhood jockeying for position at the Thanksgiving, Christmas, and Easter tables to make sure I was seated next to her. Her beauty, kindness, and sweetness glowed as bright as her namesake. Because she had no underlying health problems, I felt sure the fifty-fifty chance of survival the doctors had given her the day before my mastectomy was just a big mistake. I went into surgery certain that she'd pull through.

I wasn't really able to emotionally comprehend or process Sunny's death while I was on major narcotics for pain. I didn't even cry until five days later at her funeral. It's amazing how narcotics keep emotions at bay. I know that's why so many people get hooked on them, because they keep you free from painful emotions. Many years ago, I committed to a sober life, in large part because I welcome the full range of emotions life offers—even emotions that occasionally throw me into therapy. Feeling emotionally numb during this difficult time was strange, but I absolutely needed the pain medications.

To get to Sunny's funeral, I needed to have my hair shampooed, and that's an impossible task for me on my own because my arm movement is extremely limited. Wade drove me the half block to my hairdresser for a shampoo. I felt like I was going to puke during the entire half-block drive. It was a miserable experience, but I was determined to get to the funeral. I felt so dejected to have to stay home instead of being with my relatives who all gathered at my cousin Melissa's house to mourn her sister over a period of several days.

Seeing Sunny's children, Kelsey and Alec, both in their twenties, lose a parent conjured up some of the emotions of losing my father so long ago. I kept thinking that I'm the one who should have died, not Sunny. After all, I'm the one who has been so sick. She will be missed, and her sweetness will live on in all who knew her. I could go on and on about what a wonderful person the world has lost.

The post-mastectomy pain management has been much more challenging than it was after any of my other surgeries. Even in the hospital, I needed the nurses to deliver the IV medication hourly. In massive pain, I would call the nurse on the hour—but later, a nurse admitted that they'd been fifteen to thirty minutes late with nearly every dose. Not only was I in pain, but my chest was so tight that it felt like someone was sitting on it.

Back home, I took oxycodone for the first week and was so happy to switch back to Vicodin, because I'd been having a lot of tummy trouble. Last Saturday morning, I felt so good that I decided to meet some friends for breakfast with Wade and the kids. The car ride was short but miserable. Breakfast was fun, but I paid for it the rest of the day by throwing it up. By Sunday, I cut back to half the Vicodin, and it's been doing the trick ever since. I hope to go down to a one-quarter dosage in the next day or two.

The words of the breast surgeon at our first consultation keep coming back to me: "You're going to feel like you've been hit by a truck for the first two weeks." That's a very accurate description. I'm happy I didn't choose the lat flap; I can't imagine having stitches and pain on my back as well as my chest. There are no exercises to do yet, other than walking, and I'm not allowed to "get red in the face" when I walk. It's difficult to avoid using my pectoral muscles, which still causes pain. Simple things like opening a childproof bottle of medicine, reaching for a jar in the fridge, and buttoning a pair of jeans all engage those muscles. The pain isn't really sharp; it feels more like I have a badly pulled pectoral muscle. It also feels like there are pins and needles where the stitches are, and I have dull aches all over my chest. Riding in the car is the worst. The jostling from snow ruts and potholes is painful and leaves me very sore. I'll avoid the car until my next follow-up with the doctor.

I've yet to look at my chest. Wade has been checking the stitches daily for signs of infection, and he thinks I'll be happy with the results so far. I've seen enough reconstructed women that I have a pretty good idea of what I look like, but for some reason, I'm just not interested in seeing for myself. Of course, I've looked down with my clothes on, and they do look similar in size to my old chest, but flattened, like I'm wearing a sports bra.

On Tuesday, another very sad event happened. Our old orange kitty Rocko, a.k.a. Dr. Rocko, didn't seem to be venturing into the living room or bedrooms very much. He's normally quite social, so this was strange.

Sometimes he'll hang out in the basement, but lately he's been doing much more hiding than his normal feline introversion. So Wade and Vivian took him to the vet, who diagnosed cancer in his ribs and intestines. They immediately put him down, because the vet said he was in pain and wouldn't ultimately survive any treatment. This is the first pet Wade or Vivian has ever lost, and they took it especially hard. Rocko lived a good, long life for a cat—we got him as a stray fifteen years ago, and at the time, the vet estimated he was four or five. I'm so grateful that his suffering was short and we enjoyed so many years with our first "baby."

Our January of misery is nearly over. We look forward to a fresh start in February. We've taken cheer from the pretty flower arrangements sent by friends and family, restaurant food delivered by friends, books and magazines dropped by the house, and many phone calls and notes. Hopefully, the next time we get such an outpouring from friends, it will be for a happy cause like a graduation or wedding!

Snowboarding Mishap
Tuesday, February 17, 2009, 10:54 a.m.

Had a surprising appointment with my lymphedema therapist yesterday. I expected a routine post-surgical follow-up and assumed I'd leave with a handful of exercises designed to improve my post-mastectomy range of motion. Instead, when she measured my arm, she determined that compression bandaging is required again. Compared with the thin compression sleeve I normally wear, the return to arm bandages made me feel totally conspicuous, once again, like a dog with an Elizabethan collar. Given the time of year, if anyone asks what happened to my arm, instead of reporting roller derby as the culprit, I think I'll blame snowboarding on icy slopes. Changing up my lymphedema lies to match the season seems as normal as changing my wardrobe to match the season.

I thought for sure I'd be back to work already, but my energy is very limited. When I overdo it by folding too much laundry or running too many errands in one day, I pay for it the next by needing to sleep all day. Going to work would take more energy than I have right now.

Sponsored by Modern Medicine

Thursday, March 12, 2009, 11:06 p.m.

As I start to wind down my first full-time, no-afternoon-catnaps week back at work, I'm feeling exhausted. We were on a social fast, especially me, after my surgery. I just didn't want to be around people. I didn't feel like writing. I was in survival mode. Now that I'm physically feeling so much better, I'm ready to be around people again. Last weekend, we were busy nearly every hour, and it was a blast. We're accepting every invitation, and for the first time in months, we're extending invitations of our own. People have been commenting that both Wade and I look good, relaxed, well rested. I've started to feel some relief from worry and anxiety. Joy is commonplace. Each day is a gift, and, like a child, I'm taking each day and living it as it unfolds rather than trying to control everything. This in-the-moment feeling is mixed with the deep realization that I am literally living on borrowed time. Each day I live is sponsored by modern medicine. I would be dead if not for the twenty-first-century physicians who've worked so hard to save my life. Knowing that, technically, I shouldn't be here makes me feel like a guest in my own life—not in a bad way—just meaning that I understand things in a different light. Everything looks new and novel, and somehow, the stakes aren't quite so high. If I screw up, it won't matter much. The feeling is likely part of the high of coming back from a tough recovery, of feeling better for the first time in six weeks.

While I do feel much better, if the Advil fades from my system, I become aware of the tightness in my chest. In addition to tightness, there's also a pinching sensation under my skin where I imagine the edges of the tissues expanders sit. The tissue expanders are like balloons made with a very thick, fillable material. They allow the plastic surgeon to stretch the skin where the mastectomy was performed. Each time I see him, Dr. Nicholson adds saline into the expanders with a long needle that fits into a one-way hole in the expander. Given how uncomfortable they are now, when I see him next week, I may tell him that the expansion is over. This means I'll have to make do with the reconstruction size I've already achieved.

Recently, I went to the eye doctor for the first time in four or five years. My vision is still perfect, and my eyes are healthy. It was a change to be at a doctor's office for pure prevention. Perfect vision is something I'll tightly grip. I love knowing that my body holds some good genetic material along with the faulty. But I still felt sorry for myself after the appointment because my eyes hurt from the dilating eye drops. So I went for a chocolate shake.

Feeling better and happy in general has been tempered with a deep realization that Wade and I are generally unlucky. I've never been superstitious or believed much in luck, but starting shortly after the diagnosis, we found it almost comical to recount all our car accidents, marital accidents, and then cancer. What's next? Since losing Sunny and Rocko, we've recently only had a few minor pieces of bad luck. Now we realize that even with bad luck, we can still be happy. And I don't mean this to sound like a pity party—we just recognize that most every accomplishment has been hard won, and we've had very few lucky breaks compared to unlucky ones. We're committed to finding the fun in life, even when it isn't easy. Tomorrow is Friday the thirteenth. I've decided that from now on, Friday the thirteenth is our lucky day. Perhaps I should buy a lottery ticket.

Thinking about luck is connected to thinking about faith. My relationship with God has changed so much in the past year, but I'm not quite sure how. Perhaps contemplating luck is my way of starting to open up that conversation with myself once again. What makes us tick? What is important in life? Who is in charge?

Last night, I finished reading *The Year of Magical Thinking* by Joan Didion. She beautifully documents the year she cares for her very ill daughter and grieves for her husband, who died suddenly. The book did little to help me address the loss of my cousin Sunny; that is still a confusion of grief. But somehow the way Didion describes the loss of her husband—the person she spent time with every day—I was reminded of the grief I feel as I lose my old self, the prediagnosis Camille. Now that it's been a year and a half since the diagnosis, I can't even clearly remember who I was before. I remember the things I did, the conversations I had, but I can't re-create how my brain worked or the thoughts that filled my days. It's much like the memory of a loved one's voice fading from our memory after years without hearing that once familiar voice.

I don't actually feel depressed right now, and I don't mean to be depressing. Just . . . reflective. Wade is upstairs laughing as he watches *Caddyshack*. We made a commitment to try to have fun, despite hard times, so guess what? I'm going to walk upstairs now and laugh.

Survivor

Tuesday, March 24, 2009, 10:26 p.m.

Friday the thirteenth didn't bring a downpour of lottery riches (you must play to win, after all), but we did have a wonderful evening with friends. Wade said he hadn't heard me laugh so hard in ages, so in that respect, it was a very lucky day.

Eighteen months ago today, I went into surgery believing that would be the end of my cancer treatment. I woke up to learn other plans were made while I'd been sleeping.

And here I am, a year and a half later, waiting for another surgery—the last stage of breast reconstruction, removing the expanders—in July. Over the last eighteen months, I've devoted most of my waking hours to treatments, recovering from treatments, managing the side effects of treatments, and racing to catch up to my life that I missed in the process. I've come to think of cancer treatment as my new hobby. It's a very time-consuming, expensive hobby, but it allows me to keep on living. Recently, a fellow survivor mentioned that she had her annual oncology appointment, and she's eight years cancer-free. Wow, eight years. And with only one oncology appointment per year. That's a goal I aspire to!

The word *survivor* is an apt description for people who've lived through trying times. Eighteen months later, I'm proud to think of myself as a survivor, sharing the good company of others who have survived trials with or without cancer. I never really thought about that word much before this experience began. In fact, it had a moderately negative connotation to me. I even avoided the television show *Survivor* at all costs, partly because tuning in to any program that might show people eating insects is just too gross to risk. But now, thinking about it within the context of the past year and a half, I understand that people will do whatever they need to do to survive. The will to live can't be underestimated. To survive, people will sacrifice dignity, inject their bodies with deadly poisons, and yes, even eat bugs. And thank goodness we do fight to survive. Maybe that's what people loved about that television show—seeing how different people reacted to these survival situations. Did they become bullies? Did they crack? Or did it bring out the best in them? Or perhaps people watched the show just to be able to say, after a long hard day of work, "Hey, at least I don't need to eat bugs to survive!" Speaking of television, mine is calling me. Good night.

Mom's Heart

Saturday, March 28, 2009, 7:21 p.m.

Yesterday started at home with packing for our spring break trip to visit Wade's parents and siblings in Iowa. It ended with me packing my mom's things at her house for her unexpected stay in the hospital.

After a bit of Iowa packing, I went to an appointment at Dr. Nicholson's office, where I received a call from a nurse, explaining my mom was admitted to the hospital with fluid in her lungs and chest. Wade and I rushed to the hospital, and I stayed with her until bedtime. She was having shortness of breath due to fluid buildup caused by two leaky heart valves.

Today, her breathing is normal again, and the medication is proving effective. She needs to stay in the hospital until Monday, when they'll do an angiogram to determine the next steps. The cardiologist said surgery is the most likely route. Now that we've had nearly thirty-six hours to process everything, I'm pretty calm. Last night was a totally different story. I missed the cardiologist's visit to her room yesterday, so I had to rely on my mom's account of what he'd said. I was left with the impression that open-heart surgery was on Monday's agenda. When I insisted the nurse call the doctor, I learned my mom wasn't remembering all the nuances, and surgery isn't scheduled for Monday but is a possibility down the road.

It's terrible to worry about someone else. Dealing with rude doctors and surly nurses is awful. Trying to suddenly learn all about heart function and dysfunction is disorienting. Now that I've had a little taste of my own medicine, so to speak, I have new respect for Wade and all he's endured during my many hospital stays. It also makes me sad that my mom has had to deal with all my cancer issues. Last night, I kept clinging to the knowledge that at least Mom isn't in pain. Poor Wade (and my mom) has had to see me in oodles of pain, throwing up, unable to walk, and stoned on narcotics. Last night, Wade told me about the many hallway conversations I couldn't hear from my bed in which he argued with nurses and doctors, fighting to explain that my pain wasn't under control or that I needed different medication.

I did a lot of crying last night. Although Mom is in her seventies, she's always been in good health. Her mom lived into her nineties. I always imagined my mom would live at least as long as Grandma did—and with advances in medicine, probably even longer. Over the last eighteen months, I've been doing so much to come to grips with my own mortality, but yesterday was the first time I was confronted with my mom's mortality. Last night was the first time that my heart understood she will die someday, and that "someday" may actually happen before her one-hundredth birthday.

So many difficult feelings are already stirred up from my cousin Sunny's death. The final word is that she died of MRSA (methicillin-resistant *Staphylococcus aureus*), an antibiotic-resistant staph infection that's sometimes referred to as a superbug in news stories. MRSA is fatal to one-third of all healthy people who contract it. It's almost always fatal for people with various risk factors she didn't have, including advanced age and compromised immune systems. She got the infection in a hospital. I was amazed that when my mom was admitted to her hospital, they swabbed her nose for MRSA. They said they do that with all new patients. In all my hospital stays, I've never been tested for MRSA—very scary stuff.

Poor Wade has been really taking his lumps lately. Last weekend, he'd planned a fun "boys" weekend in Chicago. He had to cancel because he (plus Vivian and I) came down with a terrible stomach flu. It was an awful weekend that was launched by a run around the house to locate enough barf buckets for everyone. Fortunately, it was only a twenty-four-hour bug. This week, we've been feeling sorry for ourselves because last year, our plan to spend spring break in Florida was canceled because I was in radiation. We promised Vivian we'd go this year, but that was when we'd thought I only needed one more surgery, not three more. So this year, we broke the Florida promise again—mainly because it's co-pay season, so we're broke. Come hell or high water, we're going to Florida next spring break. Despite being too poor for Florida, we still looked forward to our Iowa spring break. While it's not a beach vacation, seeing family and friends makes up for the seashells we'll miss again this year.

Vivian actually thinks Iowa is pretty glamorous, which is too cute. Jackson has been talking nonstop about cows for the past week in anticipation of the trip. I was convinced late last night that my mom landed in the hospital because we'd been feeling sorry for ourselves about visiting Iowa instead of Florida—like fate said: "Oh, so you're not happy with a weekend vacation four hours south because you want a weeklong vacation twenty-four hours south? How's about this, Scheels—let's see how you like *no* vacation at all. And here's a bucketful of worry about your mom to top it all off." Lesson learned. Living in an affluent community in an affluent country, it's easy to listen to people's stories of warm-weather getaways and feel like life is so unfair. But last night, I reminded myself that each evening, most people on this planet will go to bed hungry with inadequate shelter, yet I always have plenty of food and a beautiful, newly remodeled house. We feel like such heels for whining, even privately, about not getting a Florida vacation. In reality, our lives really are blessed.

Hopefully, Mom will be back home on Monday or Tuesday, and we'll be able to take an abbreviated trip to Iowa next weekend. In the meantime, the next two days will be busy as I keep her company at the hospital. On Monday, I'll be there to be with her during the angiogram. We have the luxury of imagining the best possible scenario right now. The cardiologist said, "She's been living with these leaky valves all her life. They got out of whack because she missed a few of her meds. Just get her back on the meds, and no harm done." So until I hear otherwise, I'm going to believe everything will be just fine.

Grow It Out

Monday, April 20, 2009, 4:18 a.m.

The last three weeks have been some of the most difficult I've ever lived. Yet I've only been to one doctor appointment for me in all that time. Mom has been in and out of the hospital twice. During her last stay, I was asked to find a transitional care unit (temporary nursing home bed) for her until her open-heart surgery this Thursday. I had little more than thirty-six hours to find a place. Thanks to some quick advice from co-workers and clergy, I toured six nursing homes in twenty-four hours. My top two choices had no available beds. Choice three ranks high in every measure on the state report cards and by the people who have experience with nursing homes, but it isn't fancy. Choice two was so posh, I'd happily visit for a vacation. Choice one is a place my mom has volunteered and was clearly the best. Hopefully, when Mom is released from the hospital after her surgery, I'll be able to get her into choice one for her rehab. It's not quite as luxurious as choice two, but it has Episcopal church services daily at 10:00 a.m., which would allow her to attend to her spiritual needs as her body heals.

Being her advocate is exhausting, but it's the only work that matters to me at the moment. Now that her physical health is stabilized, I've started the work of securing her financial health by sorting through bills, organizing her checkbook, and searching her home and safe-deposit box files for all the legal paperwork she completed years ago to designate me as her voice in the event hers fails. She's still of sound mind, but she isn't interested in paying bills, and I certainly understand how that feels.

As an only child, being responsible for her care feels overwhelming. Wade has been doing as much as he can for the kids so I can focus on her health. I've been taking a lot of time off work to advocate for her at the hospital and the nursing home.

Watching health professionals care for my mother makes me understand, once again, that really the only thing we get to take with us in the end is the kindness and love we've given to others. I've stopped asking, "Why me?" and "Why now?" and "What have we done to deserve all of this?" so I can finally pause in the moment and enjoy what's directly in front of me. In most moments, I'm able to find peace, or at least security. Looking into the future, though, fear drowns out hope. I have a long road ahead as I work to understand my mom's finances and Medicare and as I support her as she prepares for and recovers from surgery. All I can do is put one foot in front of the other and step by step complete the tasks that will bring us to a better day. I'm fortunate to be surrounded by wise people who have dealt with the same issues as they learned to care for their parents.

Dealing with my mom's health issues has given me an unexpected opportunity to connect with my three cousins Nina, Melissa, and Mike—Sunny's siblings. They've explained all that happened during the days Sunny was in the hospital, when I was unable to be present leading up to my mastectomy. In July, we'll all get together to remember Sunny, and I look forward to reliving memories of her.

In another vein, I'm finally starting to comprehend my need to care for my appearance over the past few months. The last time I saw my healing coach, several weeks after my mastectomy, I told her that rather than spending time in prayer, reading, meditation, or anything really meaningful, I longed to do my nails, improve my skin, attend to my hair. She persuaded me that self-care is its own type of spiritual experience. I'm starting to understand what she means: I need to be at a very secure place in my health to go beyond the basic measures of showering, eating, and drinking. To really care for your appearance is to be attentive to your body—noticing the feel of the skin to determine how much moisturizer is needed, gently cleansing to avoid damage to the skin, looking closely to see which colors bring out the brightness of the eyes and cheeks. Caring for my appearance has been an exercise in paying attention and attending to the moment—which, as my healing coach pointed out, really are spiritual practices. Who knew that worshiping at the altar of Estée Lauder could improve my spiritual well-being?

The additional benefit of careful attention to my appearance has been lots of compliments. My bubble was burst a few weeks ago, though. As I walked into the gym, I was greeted by a security guard standing near the front desk. As the desk attendant swiped my card, my photo popped up on the computer screen. The photo shows me years ago—minus the chemotherapy pounds, plus long hair, minus months of stress and worry. The security guard (whom I've never seen before, by the way) shouted, "You look so much better with long hair!"

I smiled and nodded my agreement as I started toward the locker room.

"You should grow your hair out again!" He shouted at my back.

Again, I just smiled sweetly and kept walking. Was I really going to take beauty advice from a frumpy, overweight rent-a-cop? He himself was one big "fashion don't," yet he was criticizing what he assumed were nothing more than my poor beauty choices. I could have taught him a lesson about keeping his trap shut by explaining that what he saw before him wasn't simply a misguided haircut but evidence of a long struggle with cancer. Instead, I chose to say nothing and use it as a reminder that you just never know what's going on with people. On my way out of the gym, the security guard was still standing at the front desk. "Grow it out!" he shouted as I exited the gym.

Mom's Surgery
Friday, April 24, 2009, 7:56 p.m.

Good news—Mom's surgery yesterday was a success. She's still in the ICU and will remain there through the weekend. This morning, she made really fast progress, but her recovery is going slow this evening. I'm still at the hospital now. I keep saying I'll go home, but I can't seem to make it to the parking ramp! She's sleeping now, though, so I really will go soon.

I want to be fresh tomorrow, when she'll hopefully be a little more aware that I'm around.

As she recovers—perhaps not as quickly as I'd like—I'm keeping in my mind the image of her feeling better and enjoying life. I'm visualizing her as more energetic than she has felt in a long time. Then she'll move into the mother-in-law apartment in our newly remodeled house, and all will be well.

Today, as I gave Mom ice chips and helped to orient her on her medication status, I realized that precancer Camille would have been totally hysterical in this situation. All my own medical experiences allowed me to help calm her by reminding her she's safe, to focus on her breath, and that God's presence surrounds us. Making sense of my illness by realizing that it equipped me to help my mom makes the past eighteen months feel less like bad luck and more like valuable training.

OK. I'm going to leave the hospital now. Really, I am . . .

Mom's Recovery

Sunday, April 26, 2009, 12:41 p.m.

As my mom recovers, rather than setting up a new CaringBridge site for her, I'm going to share her updates on this site. To better organize the journal entries, I'll divide each entry into two sections: "Just the facts" with Mom's medical updates and "Camille's perspective" with my thoughts and feelings about what's going on and any updates on my own health.

Just the facts:

Over the past forty-eight hours, Mom has received several transfusions because her hemoglobin keeps dropping. They aren't sure why, but it's likely due to the fluid imbalance they're still struggling to correct. She has too much fluid in some places and not enough in others, so she's receiving medication to pull out fluid, while she's receiving IV fluids, as well. It somehow makes sense when the nurses explain it.

On Friday night, we received a call in the middle of the night, which was really scary. They had decided to intubate her, so now the machine is breathing for her. She'll remain intubated at least through today. They're keeping her sedated while she's intubated so she'll rest. Waking up and trying to communicate will only frustrate her and expend energy that she needs to heal. I'll let you know when visitors will be useful for her.

This morning, they called to tell us that she has been experiencing atrial fibrillation—which means that instead of contracting, her atrium is fluttering. Her heart rate was up in the 130s, so they asked my permission to give her medication, stop her heart, and restart it in hopes that she'd resume a normal heart rate. The procedure was successful, and now her heart rate is steady in the 80s.

She continues to respond appropriately when they rouse her to do things like squeeze a nurse's hand. Also, she opened her eyes last night, which she hadn't been able to do on Friday. I hope to talk with the doctor the next time he's around to ask some specific questions about what we can do for her. For example, does touching her hand or talking to her provide comfort? Or does it irritate her? When she was awake and without the tube on Friday, she didn't want me holding her hand at all; she was annoyed by touch. I also want to ask the doctor how many more days she is likely to be in the ICU. Are they still concerned about the hemoglobin? What are some other common setbacks we could expect?

Camille's perspective:

I'm having a horrible time organizing my days because I want to be here if she wakes up, but I don't want to be in the way of the doctors and nurses. Her care team is excellent, and I trust the quality of care she's receiving, so I think leaving them alone is probably the best I can do for her. On the other hand, I don't want her to feel abandoned or for the nursing staff to think her family doesn't care.

Yesterday afternoon, we were told she'd be sedated through the night, so we felt free to attend Vivian's school fund-raiser. It was amazing to be out with friends and laughing, having fun. I could get really addicted to going out to have fun.

This morning, I slept in; I've been so exhausted the last few days. But going out last night restored my emotional energy. Earlier this morning, even though Mom is still sedated, I still felt this panic that I needed to hurry up and get to the hospital. It's kind of crazy to feel I need to hurry up just so I can look at her.

The hospital family waiting lounge (my location as I write this) is an earthly purgatory. People just sit quietly or talk on cell phones, saying horrifying things as they relay scary medical details to those on the other end of the call. As people walk into the room, their faces are instantly familiar, as if I've known them for years. As I talked with one woman whose mother is in very similar circumstances, I kept trying to figure out who she reminds me of, who I know who looks like her. Then I realized it's just a strange familiarity, perhaps not a recognition of her face but of her spirit—we're both in the same terrible place emotionally.

My oncologist once tried to dissuade me from talking to people in waiting rooms, because their stories can be upsetting and not helpful. This morning, my waiting-room BFF's mom was taken off the breathing tube, and she's talking and making sense. I felt instantly jealous. I want my mom to be off the tube and lucid too. The upside of ignoring my oncologist's advice is that I found out my BFF's mother doesn't remember having the tube or feeling upset during that time. It gave me hope that Mom won't remember any of her discomfort.

Today is Mom's birthday, and I feel quite sad about that. Knowing ahead of time that she'd be in the hospital for her birthday, I'd imagined having people come with Mylar balloons, flowers, and treats. However, she's only allowed the Mylar balloons, and she isn't even aware it's her birthday. I don't want to upset her by explaining she's spending her birthday in the ICU.

When I arrived at the hospital, she was being repositioned by the nurses, and I saw some expression on her face. She also increased her respiration rate, because she can take extra breaths on her own in addition to the breathing the machine was doing. The nurses explained it was probably just her reacting to being moved and not really a sign of consciousness. I realized they were right, because once they had stopped moving her, sure enough, Mom's respiration rate went back to twelve, which is what the machine does for her.

I know the rational thing for me to do is to take care of anything I can now, when she isn't aware of my presence or absence. That would be smart because then my time will be available when she really needs me. In a few days, she'll need me to encourage her to cough (to prevent pneumonia) and help her to be up and walking. So I really should get the bills paid and keep up my strength so I don't just crash once she's better. But I feel this inertia, an urge to just sit and do nothing here in the hospital waiting room. For once, I have all the time in the world to get things done, and I can't accomplish anything. Very opposite my normal personality.

My right arm is starting to be unhappy again. I hope to get in for a few lymphedema physical therapy sessions next week. I'm experiencing some cording (it feels like a tight string or cord under the skin) at my elbow. Even though the therapist showed me how to fix cording months ago, it's so disgusting to feel the cording beneath my own skin. I've been too squeamish to work at it on my own. If the therapist can at least start the process, maybe I can stop being such a big baby and work out the rest of it.

The table in the waiting room is open now; I'm going to hog the whole thing by spreading out my bills and Mom's bills and getting them paid. Thank you for your love and support during this confusing and exhausting time.

Information Overload
Monday, April 27, 2009, 4:50 p.m.

Just the facts:

Twice today I've been asked to authorize procedures to help Mom fight her way back. Once for dialysis, the other for a heart pump, which should improve her rhythm. The surgeon was hopeful when he called about the dialysis but was alarmed when he called later about the pump because an EKG showed some additional trouble that he hopes the pump will address. When I asked about her anticipated quality of life, he said he doesn't know about that because we need to see if she can survive first. He said she has a fifty-fifty chance of surviving the night. He thinks she'll make it but can't be sure. Please keep her in your prayers.

Camille's perspective:

Information overload.

Tonight
Tuesday, April 28, 2009, 12:51 a.m.

Mom died tonight surrounded by family. Her priest came to the hospital, and that was a big comfort. We all had a chance to say prayers and say good-bye. The doctor said she wouldn't make it through the night and that discontinuing life support was the most humane thing. I'm terribly sad but also reassured that we were able to abide by her wishes to avoid life-prolonging measures if they wouldn't work—as stated in the health-care directive Mom filled out before her surgery.

Thank you for all your prayers. Tonight, heaven will be celebrating a very special arrival, and her love and generosity will live on as her legacy in all who have known her.

The Holy Spirit
Tuesday, April 28, 2009, 6:22 p.m.

Your love and support continue to amaze me—and my mom's generous spirit continues to astound me. She struggled with funeral planning for her own mother, so shortly after Grandma's death, Mom made all her own plans so I wouldn't have to handle so many decisions. It's a gift and a mercy.

In case I forget to mention it with the funeral details, her notes indicate she prefers that family not wear black.

Overall, today has been heartbreaking, sad, peaceful. I feel that the Holy Spirit has been guiding my actions and the actions of others in such a positive way over the last few days. It's a great comfort. Thanks for your continued prayers.

Funeral Plans
Thursday, April 30, 2009, 6:29 a.m.

It's hard to believe that just three days ago, I thought my mom would have a difficult recovery but would still make it. Already it seems like forever ago. Mom stopped needing her body, and now I'm realizing how difficult it is for those left behind to care for our bodies. Yesterday was the first day in many that I've eaten lunch. People have been bringing dinner and inviting us to dinner, so that meal is pretty easy to remember. Even breakfast keeps getting pushed later and later into the day. Normally, I wouldn't dream of leaving the house without makeup (or at least time allocated to apply it in the car—at stoplights, of course), but the past few days, I've been running around with a bare-naked face.

Wade's sister Carlene generously dropped everything to fly here and care for our kids and our house. It hasn't been so clean since Easter, and the kids are enjoying the rare treat of time with their auntie.

It's all the little things that send me to tears—choosing her clothes for the funeral, trying to decide what to do with the shoes I bought her while she was in the nursing home. She loved them so much. (Why didn't I buy her shoes a long time ago? I'd bought her clothes before; why never shoes?) So should I bury them with her or leave them for next year when Vivian will fit into them? What about all the get-well cards people sent after her surgery that are still in the envelopes, waiting for her to open them?

The emotions of this loss are all over the map—sadness, heartbreak, joy, peace. The most difficult is guilt. I knew that I needed Wade at my doctors' appointments because between the two of us, we could barely keep track of everything. We should have known to start going to my mom's medical appointments a long time ago. I didn't know swollen ankles and fatigue were symptoms of heart failure, but I should have called her doctor when they kept saying it was her arthritis causing the swollen ankles. When she kept icing her ankles with no results, I should have intervened. Yes, I've been busy in the past year and a half, but still . . .

I also feel guilty about using her bathroom. Here's what I mean—we moved as fast as we could to complete our upstairs before my January mastectomy. We moved into our new upstairs two days before my mastectomy. When I started feeling better in late March, in preparation for my mom moving in with us, Wade moved all our things out of my mom's two rooms downstairs. He did his part, but I failed to move my things out of the downstairs bathroom and just continued showering and dressing there each morning. It was nice to have my own bathroom. But was I somehow not making room for her in our house by continuing to use it? Did the universe send out some kind of chi, giving the message to her heart? Wade thinks it's silly to blame myself, but I guess it's all part of the grieving package.

The kids are doing OK. Thank goodness there's a great social worker at Vivian's school; she already helped us so much during my cancer treatments. Yesterday, she met with Vivian, who has started wearing the cross necklace Grandma gave her for her birthday in January—she's worn it before, but now she's wearing it nonstop. Last night, my friend Alison offered us tickets to *Legally Blonde: The Musical*, and despite my initial hesitation, we decided to attend. During intermission, Vivian and I were alone, saying how nice it was for Alison to take us to the show. When I said how nice my friend is, Vivian said, "Like Grandma." So I know she's thinking about my mom. She has cried, and so has Jackson.

When my cousin Sunny died and when our cat Rocko died, I think Jackson figured out that death means the person or animal is indeed gone. He will turn three soon after the funeral, so we'll have some kind of party for him. The day of my mom's surgery, I'd stopped by the toy train store near our house and bought some birthday gifts for Jackson—one from

Wade and me and one from my mom, because I knew she'd be still be too unwell to shop for his birthday. But giving him a gift "from Grandma" would confuse him, so now it will just be from Wade and me. I know I'll be a wreck when he opens those little trains that I intended to show to her before his party to make sure she approved.

I'm haunted by last Friday, when my mom was doing so well that she was extubated and therefore able to talk. She was delirious from the anesthesia and pain medication but still able to tell the nurse the current year and her date of birth. Mostly she talked about God and scripture. At one point, she kept asking for Matthew, and I couldn't figure out what she meant. I thought she meant a person and wondered if there was something from her past I didn't know. Eventually I figured out she wanted me to read Matthew 6:34, the passage the hospital chaplain had read to us the first time she was in the hospital. I should have known then that she was slipping away, but the doctors were so sure, up until the evening of her death, that she'd fully recover.

Now that the funeral is almost completely planned, I've started attending to Mom's financial matters. It's frustrating—and frightening—because now we have to manage our mortgage and her mortgage. Wade and I will inventory her safe-deposit box this morning and collect a few final things from her house that we'll need for the funeral. I can't imagine having the strength to sort through the objects in her house, let alone get it ready to sell, but I guess the courage will come in time; it always somehow does.

Mom's Visitation

Monday, May 4, 2009, 7:18 a.m.

Yesterday was a beautiful day. It was fun to see my friends and Mom's friends, some of whom I haven't seen for years. The atmosphere at the visitation was more joyful than sad. All day, I felt like the worst was behind me and in front of me—but for just that one day, there were very few tears, mostly happiness and pride about all Mom accomplished in her life.

Carlene, Wade's sister, once again lightened our load considerably by coming from Brooklyn to help out with our kids and the house. Just before she left, Wade's brother Mark, his wife, Barb, and their kids, Amanda and Andrew, arrived from Iowa to do the same. It was a great way for Vivian and Jackson to connect with family during this difficult time. I'll be forever grateful for their generosity of helping out in such a meaningful way. It allowed me to give Vivian the option of attending her biggest Swedish dance performance of the year. It's a dance group Mom introduced us to in the first place. Mom would have been so happy to know that Vivian got to have her performance.

After the visitation yesterday, Melissa and Uri hosted a dinner, and everyone shared memories. I shared documents about our grandpa and great-grandpa that I found in Mom's safe-deposit box a few days ago. Her safe-deposit box was like finding a pirate treasure chest, complete with jewelry, coins (from my childhood coin collection), and treasure maps to Mom's heart in the form of the things she found most precious, including cards people sent when she was born and when I was born, her nursing licenses, her Befriender (church lay ministry) training certificates. It was like finding a concise history of her entire life.

I think today's funeral will be more difficult than yesterday's visitation. We'll hear the scripture readings and hymns she selected years ago for her funeral. Normally, singing in church brings my emotions right to the surface. I'll often cry tears of joy or sadness or whatever has been in my heart during the previous week. It's always been a safe place for me to express true emotion.

At one point at the visitation yesterday, Vivian, Jackson, and their friends were running through the funeral home—Mom would have loved to see their joy and playfulness. I can't help but cry now at the thought of saying good-bye to her body later today. I'm comforted to know that she is now alive in the embrace of heaven, clothed in the peace that passes all understanding. Those who knew her will be honoring the memory of her beautiful life as they live on to act, as she did, with kindness, generosity, tolerance, love, and acceptance.

Finding Treasures

Sunday, May 10, 2009, 7:11 p.m.

I feel so totally disoriented. At any given moment, I don't know the day or the date. I don't know how many days or weeks it's been since Mom died. Everything is a jumble. Time has stood still; it has moved slowly at times and quickly at times. I keep remembering that in *The Year of Magical Thinking*, Joan Didion kept going over the time line of when everything happened. I have a new understanding of that now. And yet, I can't keep track of anything.

We've found more evidence that Mom wasn't feeling well for quite some time. As we sort through her house, I'm finding little notes and doctors' reminders. She'd been tracking her weight for years, which is something people with heart trouble know to do (sudden weight gain of three or more pounds in one day can indicate fluid retention). I'm so incredibly sad that we didn't fully know what was going on with her. My regret is overwhelming.

When Mom first died, there were concrete tasks to accomplish—plan the funeral, spend time with out-of-town guests, attend various gatherings, start sorting through her finances and house. I was all business, feeling down but getting things done. Today, I've hit a wall. I can't imagine ever going back to my office because my brain can't even comprehend what day or date it is, so how can I possibly schedule appointments with clients and then actually show up at the right place at the right time? I'm operating on pure faith that my confusion will subside soon, because I plan to return to the office next week.

The funeral was lovely. The hymns caused me only a few tears—but when they wheeled the casket into the hearse, I nearly lost my mind crying. I felt like she was being taken away from me forever. This was totally irrational because we were going to the burial afterward, so I knew I'd have one last chance to see the casket. And it was irrational because I know she'll live on in me and the others who knew her. It was even more irrational because she was already gone when she died. I'm starting to comprehend all I've lost in her. Even when I remember all the things about her that really annoyed me, I recall them with great tenderness.

Back at her house, it's comforting because it feels as if she's in the room with us as we sort through her things. By yesterday, though, it started to get more difficult. Her house doesn't look much like her house anymore because we've moved so much stuff around. I really want to be done with the sorting—but I never want to be done. Then she'll really be gone.

We've found mystery items that we'll never know what they are or how they got in her house. A bleached-blonde lock of baby hair—which baby is this from? A Nazi flag and medal—was it a war souvenir brought back from the war by my dad? Probably not, because I think all his army work was intelligence done stateside from Washington, DC. Or was it from her ex-husband? He was on a navy aircraft carrier, so maybe he brought them home? We'll never know. Several times I've found something mysterious and thought, *I'll have to ask my mom.* Then I remember that I can't.

Mom and I were a pair; it was always just the two of us against the world. Without a spouse on her part or siblings on my part, we made a complete team, and now I'm realizing that I've lost a part of myself.

I need strength to get back to everyday life. I have no idea how that will happen, but I'll continue to live in faith that eventually I'll find a way as I've done so many times before.

Back at Work

Thursday, May 28, 2009, 10:04 p.m.

The first morning back at work was really difficult. As I drove Jackson to school, I was remembering the phone call from Mom's doctor I'd received the last time I was on my way to work. I remembered crying in the office conference room as he and the cardiologist explained things weren't going well. My first morning back to work, I started crying as I arrived and then walked past that conference room, remembering how awful it was the last time I was there.

Once I started getting back into the work itself, though, I've been happy to be back. It's the perfect distraction, plus I feel good about doing something to help the community each day through my work.

I still have a cry every few days. It's hard to sleep. All I want to do is work at work and then sort things at my mom's house. We found someone to do the estate sale, and it's a huge relief to have the time frame set for that. We'll turn the house over to the estate sale company in two weeks, and the sale will be on Father's Day weekend. Then we'll work to get her house ready to list. I feel tremendous pressure to get it on the market when the weather is nice, because the market dries up considerably once it's cold outside.

Wade just brought me some ice cream, and *The Daily Show* has already started. The couch is calling, and I'm being drawn there like a magnet . . .

Shu Shu Sam of Siam

Wednesday, June 3, 2009, 7:02 a.m.

Instead of waiting for something nice to happen, our family went out yesterday and made something nice happen—the nicest thing we could possibly imagine, in fact. We went out and got a kitten! He's a six-week-old Siamese, and his name is Shu Shu Sam of Siam. The name was a collaboration that started out with his little white paws—on the way home from the humane society, Vivian was thinking of naming him Snowshoe, and then we were passing by the train yard on the way, and Jackson said, "Choo choo!" But we thought he was saying *shu shu* as a short form of *snowshoe*, and it stuck. Sam is just a name Vivian liked. After we got home, Wade googled "shu shu" and we learned that it means *uncle* in Chinese. So we unwittingly named him Uncle Sam of Siam. He's one and a half pounds of pure sweetness. He has chocolate points at his nose, ears, and tail with those little white paws. He's sleeping on Vivian's lap right now. He's just darling. Our dog, Savannah, is quite curious about him, but our big white cat, Cedric, isn't so sure about having a baby brother. Mom, a lifelong "cat lady," would have loved this tiny kitten man.

A friend told me something really wise. Her mom died ten years ago, and she still has times when she'll think, *I need to tell Mom; she'll just love this*. She said that her relationship with her mom has continued to change in the years since her mom's death. I've already experienced this a little bit by wanting to call my mom and tell her all about Shu Shu.

Today, I'll see my plastic surgeon, Dr. Nicholson. Last week, I found a bump on my right breast, and then I found three more a few days later. They're all on one line, though, and when I talked to my surgeon's partner, he told me it's probably stitches from the AlloDerm (the donor skin under the skin of my right breast). I felt reassured, but I'm still looking forward to Dr. Nicholson actually looking at the bumps and telling me it's nothing.

Grief Personified
Thursday, June 11, 2009, 7:59 p.m.

Last night, I met my grief face-to-face. It happened in a dream. I was outside my house (my life, in the language of dreams). It was a one-story house with a huge basement, which I think represents that part of my life that feels "beneath the surface" or "underground" or "buried." Anyway, I was out in the side yard looking at all our trees. Wade was in the backyard. I went into the front yard and noticed there weren't any trees, so I started thinking about adding more trees (this represents my need to be busy and distracted). Then I looked over by the side of the house, and this guy—an average, nerdy, sad sack of a guy—was greasing around in our yard. I ran to the backyard to tell Wade that someone was in our yard and to get the guy out. This pathetic guy was my grief personified. In the dream, Wade thought the guy was harmless, no big deal (to people outside of myself, my grief is manageable, but to me it feels unmanageable). Finally, Wade did help me chase the creepy sad sack out of the yard. Even the car he drove off in was pathetic—a red economy type of car, like one of those old Volkswagen Rabbits or an old Chevy Vega. I memorized the license plate, because I wanted to call the cops so they could go after him, representing my feeling that all my grief is so unfair it's criminal.

After I woke up and realized what the dream was really about, I guess I can take the same stance that Wade had in my dream—the grief isn't really all that threatening, but it's creepy and unwelcome. I know I need to spend some time grieving, but it's easier to just keep really busy.

Update on the breast bumps—yes, they were just stitches, nothing to worry about. Dr. Nicholson will take them out on July 23, when the expanders will be removed and the implants will be installed. I can't believe it's less than six weeks away. I'm so excited to have the uncomfortable expanders out. My surgeon needs to know if I want silicone or saline implants. He mostly does silicone, which is technically safe, but I have some reservations—if they rupture, it's very hard to tell. However, if saline implants rupture, you go flat immediately so it's obvious. The big drawback of saline is that the rupture rate is much higher, so the odds of needing surgery again years down the road increases. But silicone gives me the creeps. However, with silicone, I could sleep on my stomach—something I haven't done since the mastectomy. I'll spend another few weeks wrestling with the silicone-versus-saline decision.

One Day at a Time

Tuesday, June 16, 2009, 10:09 p.m.

To fight depression, my psychologist says I should be writing and spending quiet time in nature, but I don't want to do these things. I just would rather avoid my feelings at the moment.

My silicone-versus-saline dilemma has reached a tipping point. I've talked to three different women who chose saline but later switched to silicone. I'm 99 percent sure it's going to be silicone, and I'm already dreaming of being able to sleep on my stomach.

I guess it's back to one day at a time for me, which is a good way to live in the summer. No need for big plans when the weather is nice. It's better to just drift along and see where the day evolves.

Stolen Signs

Sunday, June 28, 2009, 8:52 p.m.

Last weekend was miserable. I was stressed about the estate sale. Luckily, we didn't even need to be at the sale. My sleep continues to be a precious few hours every night. Knowing that sleep deprivation is an interrogation technique used to break down prisoners, I keep wondering what I'm trying to get myself to admit by sleeping so little. I'm really missing my mom and feeling sad. I started getting a fever and was emotionally out of control—yelling at the kids, mad at Wade for no reason. Mostly I was mad at myself, feeling like this life just isn't worth living any longer.

My dark mood culminated on Sunday night when I asked Wade to call the estate sellers to find out how the sale went. Not well. Mom's house is difficult to find because it's in a development of twisty-turny streets. Even if you have directions, it's hard to find. So the estate-sale organizer wisely put up a bunch of signs. At some point in the sale, someone stole all the signs. Then someone claiming to be the president of the homeowners association started hassling him, saying sales aren't allowed. While we got rid of quite a bit of stuff, it wasn't a very profitable sale. Potential buyers had to keep calling for directions, and I assume many people gave up trying to find the house. I can't believe anyone could be so mean to remove estate sale signs—I feel like they're saying, "Here's someone who's had a loss; what can we do to make it worse?"

I calmed down during the following week but then got sick with a high fever for two days. My doctor told me to rest for two days. I'm worried about being healthy enough for my July 23 surgery.

This weekend threatened to be a bad one, as well. We'd planned a trip to Iowa but canceled when Vivian awoke throwing up on Friday morning, and she continued into the evening. She was still sick yesterday morning but thankfully recovered by the afternoon.

As it turned out, it was a relief to have a no-obligations weekend. It's been months since we've had this much free time. We went to a party on Saturday night, and then we went to the neighbor's house where the kids played. Today, I took Vivian and her friends to a movie, and we had neighbors over for dinner. I made a long shopping trip to Target yesterday for the first time in months. It felt like a normal weekend. And after five days of allergy medicine and several nights of sleep, I feel like a new person. Having a relaxing weekend was just what the doctor ordered.

A quick Shu Shu update—he has doubled in weight and in cuteness. We love our little man.

Silicone

Monday, July 20, 2009, 10:16 p.m.

Only three days until my final surgery! It's always a bit nerve-racking to anticipate being put under, but at least this time it's purely for aesthetic reasons. I don't have to worry about the doctor discovering cancer when I'm on the table. The surgeon will remove the tissue expanders and replace them with silicone breast implants. Yes, I decided on silicone.

After the implants are in, I'll need to wear a bra for three weeks to help some of the stitches heal. It will be weird to wear a bra again, because I haven't needed one since January. Then after three weeks, I can throw the bra away and never wear one again. Truly, this is the silver lining of the whole experience!

A while back, I was considering getting a little liposuction and maybe a tummy tuck along with this surgery. It would cost big bucks out of pocket. Dr. Nicholson talked me out of it. He said that because I'm only just over one year out of chemo, I should give myself another year to get my metabolism back.

That's one thing I learned after completing chemo—the kind I had makes it nearly impossible to lose weight for two years after ending the treatment. Plus, once I do lose weight, it will show up in different places than it did before. For example, instead of just having a little pooch below my belly button, now I grow fat clear up to my sternum. This is partly menopause and partly the tamoxifen, which is an androgen. So essentially my body is looking less feminine from a lack of estrogen. My surgeon said that after I start to lose weight, then we can talk, but he doesn't think I'll need any additional plastic surgery once the pounds "start melting off" (his prediction). I hope he's right!

I'm so excited to get these tissue expanders removed. They're really uncomfortable. They look weird too—fine with clothes on, but when I look in the mirror without a shirt, they are really uneven. My plastic surgeon said that's because one of the expanders turned, which sounds pretty creepy. But not as creepy as more cancer, so I'll deal with it. Tissue expanders are like being pregnant. Once you get close to your "due date," all you want is to get that thing—expander or baby, whichever the case may be—out of your body.

My mental health has been pretty good in the past two weeks. However, before that, I was sinking pretty low. There were many days that I couldn't see the value in continuing to live this life. Were it not for Vivian already having so many losses, it would have been pretty easy for me to just let go of this life. While I'm too chicken to ever actually cause myself harm, I have considered simply running away. Even in my dreams. In one memorable dream, I went on a totally optional work trip over Wade's birthday weekend. In another, our entire family moved to Wade's home-town in Iowa on a whim.

Two weekends ago, I took a break from working nearly every waking moment and spent some time with friends and family. I was like a new person by Monday. It's amazing what a little rest and recreation can do for one's mental health.

That being said, it's hard to commit to rest when there's just so much work to do. We've organized everything from my mom's house into one of the two rooms of the mother-in-law apartment we created for her at our house. The other room we're making into a guest room. My mother-in-law will use it when she comes to help Wade with the kids during my expander surgery and the day after.

Wade is nearly done painting my mom's entire house as we prepare to sell it. He's also swapping out three sinks, and two of the bathrooms need new vanities and countertops. He's already replaced all the kitchen and dining room flooring, and the carpet guys are coming tomorrow to do the rest of the house. We really want to get it on the market yet this summer, so poor Wade will, in addition to his day job, have to keep working there most afternoons.

Having experienced my mom's death, as I prepare for this surgery, I feel so in touch with my mortality. Not in a morbid way, but now sometimes I'll look down at a piece of my jewelry and think, *Someday, Vivian will look at this after I'm gone and remember that I wore it.* Or I'll look at my clothes in the closet and know that someday they'll be bagged up for charity.

My mom used to always talk about "when I die, you need to do (this or that)." I never wanted to listen. I would literally put my hands over my ears. I thought it was morbid and scary. Now I realize that death is a natural part of the human experience. It's a gift to be in touch with my mortality because many of life's confusions result from not knowing what's important. Now I know that kindness, comfort, and love are the only things that really count in this life. I wish I would've been more in touch with Mom's mortality before she died. I really thought she'd never die. Isn't that crazy? Now I'm trying to grasp that everyone around me will one day be gone—and I should treat them and our time together as precious. Coming to terms with mortality in a culture that doesn't like to acknowledge it feels like a private journey. It's impolite to discuss death in everyday conversation. It's difficult to articulate feelings we rarely consider. So while I'm happy to have this new awareness, I'm not sure what exactly to do with it.

A darling little kitten just jumped into my lap, so maybe that's what my spirit needs in this moment.

The Final Surgery
Sunday, August 2, 2009, 4:53 p.m.

The surgery to end all surgeries is over! The first two days afterward, I was so miserable that I was cursing my decision to reconstruct. Why didn't I just go flat? The Vicodin was upsetting my stomach to the point that I gave up taking it less than forty-eight hours after surgery. That was possible, in part, because the pain was nothing like the mastectomy pain. The next forty-eight hours weren't much better, except that I was able to focus on reading magazines. Being able to eat and keep it down was also a happy experience. A week out from surgery, I was still grumpy and feeling bored but able to handle the pain. Now it's just a matter of getting my energy up, which I'll work on in the next week.

A funny thing happened on the way to the operating room. The nurse brought me into an exam room, handed me a plush terry robe, and asked me to undress. When I was done undressing, I snooped around, noticing the usual stuff—lights, clean linens, silk thread for stitches. Then I noticed a big black bottle exclaiming the word "Toxins" and—I kid you not—a skull and crossbones. I wish I had a picture of it. It was so funny. Then I spied something as frightening as it was funny a full-color poster that said—again, I kid you not—"Only WE can prevent surgical fires." Under that headline was a quote from Dr. Nicholson: "Nurses and staff are empowered to speak up if they notice an element is left out of the holster." Between the words was a photo of a surgical scene: a patient covered in blue sheets with a fire raging on one of the sheets! A new worry to add to the list—surgical fires! When I asked the nurse about it, she said the sign refers to a heating element they use to cauterize tissue. What I didn't ask was why my surgeon had a poster made about it. Did he become aware of this issue at some conference and he was being proactive? Or did he learn about surgical fires the hard way? Sitting there, waiting for surgery to begin, I had a choice—laugh or cry. I chose laughter.

When I awoke from surgery, I experienced the familiar postsurgical "I'm alive!" euphoria. I'm so happy to know this is the final surgery. I need to remind myself that there may be other things in the future. But this is the last in this series—the last for the foreseeable future, anyway. My excitement at being "done" with all my medical treatments is tempered by fear of a new cancer occurring, or even worse, the old one coming back and metastasizing.

At the dentist a few weeks ago, they offered me a new screening for oral cancer. I hesitated before consenting to the screening—if I have oral cancer, do I really want to know? They did the screening and it was negative. Whew.

This whole final surgery experience made me miss my mom even more. We've had so many firsts since her death—first Mother's Day without her, our first wedding anniversary (our fifteenth) without her, and my first surgery without her. Later this week is my fortieth birthday—my first birthday without her. We'll celebrate with just our little family on my actual birthday, and then we'll have a bigger party sometime later this month. We'll be celebrating so many things—fifteen years of marriage in July, my fortieth birthday in August, and two years cancer-free in September.

Out of Control

Thursday, August 13, 2009, 5:54 a.m.

After my last post, things started spinning out of control—Wade cut his thumb on his table saw while working at my mom's house. It took eleven stitches to reattach the tip, which was nearly cut completely off. The next day, Vivian was having chest pain, so I took her to urgent care—turned out to be residual from a cold she'd had earlier in the week, which isn't uncommon for kids her age, but it was scary because they did an EKG and chest X ray just to be safe. In the midst of it all, we found out that the house across the street from my mom's is going on the market—not good news for us, because it will drive down our selling price.

All of these things in combination started me thinking that this life isn't worth living, which is a terrible thing to think when I've fought so hard for my life. Being so busy with our lives and settling my mom's affairs is already a lot—having anything extra to manage nearly pushes me over the edge.

Then I was back to work on Monday, and suddenly, life started to seem more normal and manageable. While it's always super busy getting caught up at work, it's such a stabilizing factor that my mental health improves dramatically in short order. It provides a positive focus and forces me to get outside of my head.

Clarity
Thursday, August 20, 2009, 9:36 p.m.

Mom's house has had a few private showings this week, and the open house was well attended on Sunday. If we can sell it by February, I'll be thrilled. In this market, it's impossible to predict much of anything, but at least we're off to a good start.

On Sunday at church, I had a moment of clarity at the Communion rail. I often feel a sense of gratitude as I walk past the choir toward the altar. If I have one of my kids with me, I sometimes quiz them, "Do you know why we're doing this?" Then I remind them that it's to remember Jesus and what a huge sacrifice he and God have made for us. As I approached the railing this week, I realized that I was sharing the Communion experience with individuals who've given away millions of dollars of personal wealth to charity, alongside individuals who need to accept charity to survive. God doesn't care about any of that. How much we have or don't have doesn't matter at all. We're all equal as we make our way back to the pews.

We're also equal in God's eyes regardless of our good or poor health. Only the health of our souls matter to him. The health of the body and the wealth of the individual are both just distractions. I felt my soul being cleansed by the water of the Spirit as I realized that in this moment, I am alive, I am safe, and I am comfortable, loved, and free. What more could I possibly desire?

Lighter
Friday, August 28, 2009, 8:12 p.m.

The other day, a perceptive friend said, "You look lighter."

My reply: "Well, I recently lost a pound—"

"No," she said, "your spirit is lighter."

Finally, understanding her remark, I replied, "Yes, in fact, I feel like twenty pounds has been lifted. We sold my mom's house after only ten days on the market!"

And it's true; just four months after she died, we're relieved to have a buyer for Mom's house. It's a young couple who love the place and will hopefully have a very happy life there. Wade did so much hard work to make it look fabulous. While we won't get rich off the deal, it's a huge relief to know we won't go broke paying two mortgages. It's difficult to say good-bye to the place, but the memories will always live on.

My birthday party last weekend was just as I'd imagined it—kids playing on the backyard swing set, grown-ups chatting and chilling. We had about fifty adults and thirty kids—the biggest gathering we've ever hosted at our house. After our guests left, Wade said, "Let's do that again soon!" I loved having something happy to celebrate. In lieu of birthday gifts, we also raised a good amount of money for the American Cancer Society—we'll be sending a $400 donation this week.

I've also been enjoying time with the kids. We have the piano from Mom's house—it's a player piano, so Vivian and I have been singing along to all these old songs from the 1920s, '30s, and '40s. Some of them I sang to her when she was little, others she's never heard, and yet she somehow knows the tunes even the first time she sings them. She really is an old soul. Tonight, Jackson attended the first birthday party he's been invited to attend sans Vivian. He had a blast.

This will be my last post in this CaringBridge blog. It's bittersweet. While there will be tests, scans, and probably some scares in the future, the most intense part of this journey is in the rearview mirror. It's amazing how much easier life is without another test result, surgery, or chemo around the corner. I'll miss all the support and love you've given me with your kind wishes here on CaringBridge, by e-mail, and in person. The rest of my life will be calmer knowing that if something really bad ever happens, I have a community nearby to break the fall. I hope that's something you've learned from following my journey—that if you ever suffer from some unexpected twist in life, people will show up in more ways than you can possibly imagine.

To say good-bye, I'd like to share something I've been thinking about lately: inheritance. As we negotiated the details of selling Mom's house, I fretted over money. Quickly, I realized that money is not my inheritance.

My legacy from my mother is her kindness, her love, her passion for education, her faith, and her ability to laugh even when the going gets tough. The Bible talks again and again about inheritance. These are the things we are given by God the Father—gifts we don't earn but receive by simply being God's children. Knowing that one day I'll claim my true inheritance in the kingdom of heaven calms my fears and colors my days with hope.

Thank you for being my home, my fortress during my cancer journey. Thank you for reading all these postcards from Camp Chemo. My wish for you is love and hope for all your days and nights. May peace be with you always.

metastasis

Returning to Camp

It's Back...

Thursday, April 5, 2012, 5:42 p.m.

I closed out this CaringBridge site over two years ago, but I'm sorry to report that I need to open it up again. My first postcard now that I'm back at Camp Chemo should read, "Wish I Weren't Here..."

Here's how it all happened. I've been seeing an orthopedist, Dr. Smith, for pain that started last summer in my hip. Pain so bad it's made me limp. Lately, the only way I can walk is with crutches. For all these months, I thought it was because my gait had changed after a bunion removal surgery in January 2011.

A few weeks ago, Dr. Smith ordered an MRI and called late that same night to explain the MRI revealed the breast cancer has metastasized to my bones—hips, pelvis, scapula, femur, ribs, and spine. The hip, my main site of pain, showed the most cancer.

After the phone call, Wade and I cried like babies. Wade threw up twice. Luckily, the kids were asleep, and we were able to face this news like children but sans children.

Since then, I've been to a doctor at least once every day—CT/PET scan, bone biopsy, radiation oncologist, regular oncologist, and daily radiation starting yesterday.

The good news is that the cancer isn't in any soft tissue, and it's still estrogen receptive. That means treatment will include daily pill of an aromatase inhibitor to block any remaining estrogen. I'll receive daily radiation to my hip for a few weeks. They can't radiate all the bones, just the most painful ones to try to decrease the pain.

We don't have a prognosis yet, but my oncologist, Dr. Anderson, said he hopes my life will be measured by years and not by months. However, because this is metastatic breast cancer, a.k.a. terminal, or Stage IV, we aren't able to hope for a cure. They will extend my life as long as possible and keep me comfortable as long as possible.

Over the last week, Wade and I have looped in a small number of friends and family. We wanted to keep mum with the kids at first. Tonight, we spoke with each kid individually. It was awful, especially with Vivian. She still has painful memories of my first diagnosis and my arduous treatment. We're only talking with the kids about my treatment. We won't discuss end-of-life issues until we get more information about when that might come. We want to allow the kids to express their fears and emotions to us and other adults who are important to them, but we don't want to burden them with information that will only cause more stress.

My mantra now is "Keep Calm and Carry On," which is based on World War II British Ministry of War posters designed to boost morale. This mantra suits me, even though I sometimes dissolve into tears.

Last weekend, I started to get paperwork in order by looking into my long-term disability and life insurance. I worry about how my family will do without me. I keep thinking the more planning I can complete now, the more I can enjoy time with my family, because I'll know they'll be provided for.

We're going to have some difficult decisions in the upcoming months, but today, I have a bowlful of raspberries, a backyard full of happy little kids, and good music on the radio. So far, we're doing our best to keep calm and carry on.

You're Getting Very Sleepy . . .

Thursday, April 12, 2012, 7:43 a.m.

Sending appreciation for your guestbook messages, phone calls, e-mails, and visits over the past week—your love and care are so important.

I've had tremendous relief of pain in my hip, thanks to daily radiation. Now I'm taking 25 percent of the pain medication I had been taking, yet I'm feeling 50 percent better. The last few days I've walked around the house a little bit without a crutch, but I pay for it the next day.

The kids have been minimally curious about what's happening. After talking with a few professionals, we've decided we won't discuss the end of life until it's just around the corner. The way kids process information, if we say I will die from this, they'll think it will happen tomorrow. We were advised to wait until the end is close and the kids are able to observe big changes—like if I'm unable to eat or get out of bed. The kids appear mentally healthy, and they're fighting with each other as much as ever. We're telling friends to let us know if they hear Vivian or Jackson asking questions, because kids often don't want their parents to know they're worried.

We're still waiting for a prognosis. It should come this afternoon at our first formal meeting with Dr. Anderson (we've met with a radiation oncologist and an on-call oncologist from the practice already). We have so many questions about how metastatic breast cancer progresses and what we can do to keep me as healthy and comfortable as possible. I hope to find out what I can do to control my weight. Without being able to exercise for nearly a year, due to last year's foot surgery and then the cancer pain, I've gained close to twenty pounds. I can't afford to become diabetic, because it would limit the treatment options.

During radiation last week, I came up with an idea for how to keep the cancer from expanding. Imagining white blood cells killing cancer in a battle scene never really worked for me. I'm a mother, not a fighter. So my idea is to hypnotize the cancer cells to sleep. I'll sing them lullabies, tuck them in, walk them through a field of poppies a la *The Wizard of Oz*. I'm already doing this in my meditations. I don't really hate the cancer; it seems unhealthy to hate something in your own body. In a small way, I'm thankful for the message it keeps trying to deliver: slow down, and enjoy those close to you.

Here's a lullaby I wrote for Jackson when he was a baby, one I've been singing to the cancer cells:

It's time to go to sleep tonight,
It's time to close your little eyes,
And it's time to dream of things you like.
It's time to go to sleep.
It's time for you to go to bed,
And rest your little tiny head.
Yes, it's time to go to sleep, I said.
It's time to go to sleep.

Less News

Thursday, April 12, 2012, 8:26 p.m.

Less news is better than no news.

Saw Dr. Anderson today. We wanted him to provide a list of statistics, much as he did when I saw him for the first time four and a half years ago. We wanted to know the expected result of various treatments. Instead, he explained that the drug he hopes will work isn't even FDA approved, so they don't know how long it will provide "progression-free survival," which simply means keeping the cancer stable. It's the best he can do for us. The radiation is primarily for pain control.

When we pushed him for a prognosis, he said that if the cancer stays how it is (meaning if the treatment doesn't work), he would expect that I have two or three years. If it works, he expects six or seven years. If it moves to the soft tissue (liver and lungs are most likely), then he thinks I'd live a year or two. Really, he just doesn't know what to expect. We laypeople think medicine is an exact science, but he explained that metastatic breast cancer behaves differently in each individual.

We asked about when I'd be able to walk without a crutch and maybe even regain the ability to walk more than a few feet without resting. He thought the radiation would continue to help but that I'll never get back to the mobility I once enjoyed. He also wasn't certain the radiation would provide a long-term improvement.

He also surprised me with a one-hour IV infusion of Xgeva, a bisphosphonate used for strengthening bones. At least I got some free apple juice out of the deal. I'll have this infusion monthly, along with labs and a doctor's visit that will include two shots in my butt (hormones), and two Afinitor (chemotherapy) pills a day. The Afinitor is a new (not yet FDA-approved) medication approved by my insurance, much to everyone's surprise. Let's just say that, next to my harp, these new chemotherapy pills are the most expensive items in our entire house. I'm guessing this doesn't really put our home at risk for break-ins because experimental cancer drugs and harps are both pretty difficult to fence.

Overall, we're feeling let down about not having a definitive prognosis. No crystal ball is available, which is frustrating because I'm such a planner.

Wade and I feel sad, but we're also determined to spend time with the kids in ways they'll remember for years to come. There are several trips I wanted to take with the kids during their high school and college years, and we made a commitment today to make some of those happen within the next few years. Any delay seems like we're squandering time, so we're going to plan some adventures soon.

Jackson is upstairs giggling like a maniac, clearly not wanting to go to bed for Dad. So I'm going to snuggle the little guy and then watch *Arrested Development* (we're on our third time watching the series, and it's still funny). I still believe that sometimes, laughter is the best medicine.

Comfort

Friday, April 13, 2012, 5:12 p.m.

After the bone-medicine infusion, I've had flu-like symptoms, as predicted. And for some reason, now my hip hurts more than it has since I started radiation. Hopefully, it will settle down over the weekend.

This morning, I had the lucky opportunity to provide comfort to someone else. As I was exiting my oncology office, a woman was lying on a waiting room couch. I asked if she was OK. She said she still needed to check in, and I asked if I could do that for her, and she agreed. Then I came back and asked if I could sit with her and touch her arm while we waited, and she said yes. She was wearing a "chemo cap" (a little hat made of T-shirt material), and she looked so sick. I knew exactly how she felt—nauseous, dehydrated, exhausted. She would get fluids after her radiation treatment today, but she'd come from a town thirty miles away. Car rides are awful when you feel like that. I'm happy I was able to sit with her while she waited.

Over the past week, I've been trying to get our financial house in order. I've consolidated all our bank accounts into one and made sure Wade has access to it. This week, I'll also continue getting our actual house in order, which is a never-ending process for everyone, cancer or not.

I went back to work this week, and it was great to feel useful. Tonight, we'll go to a comedy show. Can't get enough of laughter these days.

Ghost
Sunday, April 15, 2012, 8:05 p.m.

Saturday I slept in. Even without a big to-do list, I still felt frustrated by late afternoon that not enough got done around the house. I'm someone who's been described as hyper since childhood. Now as an adult with a midwestern work ethic, it's maddening when I feel a day become a waste of time. Poor Wade wanted to get together with a friend; he needs the support, right? But I made him cancel his friend time so I could complain and cry while we sorted through junk that's been stored in our dining room buffet drawers for years—so I could feel I'd accomplished something. Such a mean wife.

I'm totally fed up with my physical exhaustion, my pain, and my inability to get around. It makes me realize I'll need to choose my activities carefully going forward. We decided to take up some friends on their generous offer to fund a cleaning service—they'll start later this week. We've never had one before—there's still something so not midwestern about allowing someone else to clean up our mess. But it's very painful for me to reach down to the ground and even to reach down to lower shelves, so cleaning is difficult and at times impossible.

You know those movies where someone encounters a terrifying ghost, freaks out, and starts to run, but then some little kid will calmly ask the ghost, "What do you want?" The ghost, it turns out, just wants to deliver a message to the living. That's how I'm thinking of this cancer: not a terrifying ghost but an inert one, trying to deliver urgent messages to me, like slow down and remember what's most important. Even so, I can't bear for the sun to go down on an unproductive day. I've been trying to thank these little cancer cells for passing along this important message, sing them to sleep, and then send them each down the river of my blood-stream. I imagine them in little reed baskets, like the baby Moses floating down the Nile. A lullaby to keep them quiet as they fall asleep and float away through my bloodstream, and then finally they'll leave my body to fight the pharaoh of the municipal sewer system.

Now that I'm getting ready to snuggle my little mister (and little cancer cells) to sleep, I'll leave you with a song that I sometimes use to put my kids to sleep. People of a certain age might recognize it from a TV variety show with an accordion-wielding host (ahem, Lawrence Welk). And a one, and a two, and a—

> *Good night, sleep tight, and pleasant dreams to you*
> *Here's a wish and a prayer that every dream comes true*
> *And now 'til we meet again*
> *Adios, au revoir, auf Wiedersehen*
> *Good night!*

Never

Monday, April 23, 2012, 9:01 p.m.

Radiation has me really, really fatigued. Tomorrow is my last day of radiation, and I hope to be more energetic within a few weeks. However, the doctor tells me I won't be as energetic as before. I'll never forget the response when I asked when I'll get my energy back: Dr. Anderson and his nurse both looked at me and shook their heads, and the doctor said, "Never."

The pain is more manageable than it was before the radiation. Prior to the diagnosis, I had been taking ten Advil, ten Tylenol, and two Percocet, plus icing my hip ten times per day and using a small electrical pain control device called a TENS (transcutaneous electrical nerve stimulation) unit four times per day. This still wasn't controlling the pain adequately. Now I'm taking just four to six Advil per day, minimal ice, some TENS unit action, and one Percocet before bed.

Overall, I'm getting around pretty well with a crutch or, on really good days, a cane. Having the pain under control is a big relief, and while the doctor couldn't guarantee that the benefit of the radiation will be long term, I'll take it for now.

As always, being back at work is helpful. Still trying to find a balance between work and enjoying time at home. It will probably take a while to figure that out. Then again, that's not a cancer thing; that's just a twenty-first-century thing.

Sometimes I feel like I'm living in opposite world: I used to go to the gym four or five nights a week and felt way more energetic and healthy when I'd go. Now the more I move, the worse I feel. It's odd to be taking the elevator instead of the stairs and reminding myself not to move too much or I'll be sore the next day.

Same goes with the narcotics. On Thursday night, I was feeling so good, I decided to forgo the Percocet before bed, and the next morning, I felt totally hungover. Weird to live in a world where *not* taking narcotics makes me feel hungover.

Friday morning, I was tired and sore, and the mouth ulcers from the Afinitor that started earlier in the week were getting so bad that eating or drinking anything was miserable. So I asked to see my nurse after radiation. She gave me a magic mouth "swish" to use before eating. It contains lidocaine, which numbs the mouth, and that has been wonderful. This nurse has known me since 2007, and she's accustomed to my perky manner. So when I came in weepy, complaining about my mouth sores and asking questions like, "If I'd had the MRI that found my cancer earlier, would my prognosis be better?" and "Did the first MRI miss something?" and generally beating myself up or looking for someone else to blame for this whole fiasco, she wanted to help. She assured me nothing could have been done differently, and then she delicately asked if I'd ever consider taking an antidepressant. My chart wasn't in front of her, so I had to explain that I'm already on more antidepressants than ever before. Even with the antidepressants, I'm constantly aware that I'm grieving my past life. I'm also mourning my expectations for the future. I guess there will be a few bad days here and there. My psychiatrist says if I cease to feel emotion, I'll know the antidepressant dose is too high. He also explained that antidepressants won't make me happy all the time and it won't make the problems go away, but it will provide more resilience to deal with whatever is happening. The fact that I can cry reassures me that the dose is just right and that I'm still part of the human race.

Most of the weekend was spent crying, sleeping, and working in our basement to conquer five hundred square feet of *Hoarders*-style bankers' boxes that we moved from my mom's house after she died. They contain about 150 years of family history that needs to be edited into a few boxes for each of my kids. But I don't quite have the emotional fortitude or energy now to sort the photos and letters dating from the 1850s to the present day.

The other motivation for purging is that Wade and I are pretty sure we're going to sell our house. Even before the diagnosis, we realized we'd been living on a budget too tight for comfort. Now that I want to travel and enjoy more time with the kids, a smaller house makes sense. My mobility issues have me sleeping in a main floor spare bedroom, because it's very difficult to make it upstairs to our bedroom. It will take months to get our house ready and maybe months to sell it, but we've already been checking out some small, one-level homes in the neighborhood.

Sunday was the best day of the weekend. During church, both kids wanted to stay with me instead of going to Sunday school. They sat on either side of me "grooming" my long, brunette hair (halfway down my back these days) braiding it and finger combing it. Jackson snuggled and lay across Vivian's lap and my lap. Being close to my little kittens is so wonderful. We're still focusing on my treatments, not the outcome, and sometimes that's difficult. Vivian and I recently watched a wedding show, and after she was in bed, I was in tears with Wade comforting me as I thought about how heartbreaking it would be if I died before her wedding. Then as we drove past a wedding shop this weekend, Vivian pointed out a wedding dress that "would be a great prom dress if it was in a different color," which also made me tear up. But maybe her prom is something I could still see? I want to be with her in person to feel her soft hair, zip up her dress, and try to scare her prom date before they leave the house. Even if I'm not around in body, I can probably do that last part pretty effectively as a ghost, right?

A Very Busy Day
Tuesday, May 1, 2012, 9:12 p.m.

Woke up around 10:30. Ate breakfast and a handful of pills around noon. Then I rested and made to-do lists. Doesn't sound busy yet, but wait—I took a shower (second one in a week), put on makeup (second time in a week), and drove myself—wait for it—a half block to the dentist. Walking that far is still too painful. Vivian went with me, so after my appointment, we walked across the street to buy May Day candy and Vivian's birthday gift for Jackson. He turns six this weekend, and his birthday list has two items: Legos and candy. Then we drove home, made May baskets (construction paper cones with ribbon handles stapled on), and I walked across the street to chat with neighbors while the kids delivered baskets to their pals. I sat at the table for dinner for the first time in days, and I even washed two pans. It's been weeks since I've washed a dish because it's been too physically demanding. After reading to Jackson, I made a snack for him, washed my face, brushed and flossed, and now I'm ready for some shut-eye. A few weeks ago, this would've been a huge failure of a day, but today it's a big success.

The other days haven't been quite so productive.

Tuesday (a week ago): Showered, took kids to school, had my final radiation treatment, went to work, went to bed early. Mouth ulcers started to get better, but eating still hurt.

Wednesday: Worked a half day. Took the afternoon off so I could rest up for book group. Had a blast with the brilliant women I've been reading and meeting with every few weeks for ten years. They are so caring and protective of me, I just love it. Back at home, I noticed some pain at the bikini line crease on my right leg. Showed Wade, and he realized it's a radiation burn. They mentioned this crease is prone to burns, but I forgot to put extra lotion on this area during treatment.

Thursday: Didn't feel well, was exhausted, and had tummy trouble. Although I hadn't showered, I pulled my hair into an updo (dirty hair is actually better for that, anyway), put on some makeup, and attended the Learning Fair at Vivian's school. She chose dark energy and dark matter as her subject. Truly, this child is an old soul. So glad to have attended, but it took all the energy of the day.

Friday: Felt worse, major tummy trouble, exhausted, low-grade fever. Napped most of the day. Mouth sores were better, so eating wasn't bad, but my entire digestive system was f*#%@ed. As soon as I ate anything, I bloated up like a balloon—unsightly and very painful. At the end of the digestive process . . . well, let's just say that number two was my number-one most dreaded activity. It's all side effects from the radiation of the pelvis. So while the visible burns are like a very bad, deep sunburn, the burns inside my body are much worse because radiation cooks like a microwave, from the inside out. The clinic gave me five different medications to address my various tummy issues, but they'll take time to work. Vivian and I meant to watch wedding-dress shows on TV and look at my Barbies, but I was only able to lie in bed and tell her about my various Barbies and their outfits. It was fun, but not exactly what I'd planned. A fever emerged that night, and I woke up soaked with sweat several times.

Saturday: Fever gone, exhausted and filthy, but a shower seemed as likely as climbing a mountain. The kids set up camp in my new ground-level bedroom. Played Legos with Jackson, napped, cried, watched TV—and finally, took a shower. Felt like I could conquer the world for a few minutes. Vivian blow-dried my hair. Ate dinner with the family only because my mother-in-law, Beckie, was in town for the night.

Sunday: Tummy still hurt, exhausted, trying to figure out what to eat was still very confusing, medicine started to help. I went outside in the backyard for a little while. My mother-in-law stayed longer than planned to help Wade with housework. A lovely thing happened—I awoke from a nap to hear loud laughter in the dining room. For a long time, I just listened to Wade, his mom, and the kids laugh, and then they'd get quiet for a minute and laugh again. It was genuine music to my ears. As an only child, I'm easily prone to feeling left out of the fun, and in my healthier years, I would've felt lonely listening to them from the other room. But I know I won't be around forever, so it helps to hear them having a great time without me, knowing they can laugh. It gives me hope that they'll be fine without me someday. After walking into the dining room, I found out they were watching funny pet videos on the computer, so I joined in the fun.

Monday: Tummy was 60 percent restored, but still exhausted. Couldn't drive the kids to school, let alone think about showering and work. Talked to my boss and HR about short-term disability. Called my oncology clinic to find out what I can expect in the upcoming weeks and months in terms of energy level. The radiation and all the pills I'm taking list "fatigue" as a side effect, but I explained that I need to do some planning for getting back to work. They'll call me later. And, as promised, for the first time ever, and thanks to some very kind friends and relatives, our house was cleaned by professionals! Everything smells lemon fresh and looks amazing. Should have done it years ago. While the house looks and smells great, me, not so much; my last shower was Saturday.

Today, Tuesday: The nurse called back and said it will be two to four more weeks before we can assess the long-term effects of the medications I'm taking. The radiation will continue to ping around in my body (and burn me inside and out) for another three weeks, and then any fatigue from radiation should ease up. So in a few weeks, we'll be able to review how I'm feeling to determine when I can go back to work and if the medication is also contributing to the fatigue. The word *fatigue* is specific, because what I feel is different from sleepy or tired. I've been napping nearly every day, but I also feel sort of weak, and I need to lie awake in bed not doing much of anything.

At this point, I'm realizing that I don't have the energy to juggle everything I want to do—healing, work, kids, home—so I might need to back off work more than I wanted. The last time around, I could predict how long I'd need off from work with each surgery (generally, one week of rest per hour in surgery) and how long I'd need after each chemo treatment. My radiation didn't really do much besides char my skin last time. This time, it's a whole different set of side effects. I hope the fatigue is from the radiation and not the medications, because I'll need to be on the medications indefinitely.

That's been my week. So much more to share, but my sleeping medication is starting to kick in, and it's best not to fight it.

Death Row

Wednesday, May 9, 2012, 9:11 p.m.

Tomorrow, I'll see Dr. Anderson, and I'm terrified. It's been ages since I was nervous to see him. Feeling this way defies logic, because I know he won't have bad news for me right away. He'll check my blood for tumor markers, and we won't know anything for at least twenty-four hours. Mostly, I hate thinking about bad news that may come (for example, the cancer has spread from my bones into my soft tissue); plus I'm worried that the chemotherapy I'm taking isn't working.

At the end of the appointment, I'll spend an hour hooked up to an IV for my bone-strengthening medicine. Hopefully, I'll get a private room and I can just hang out reading magazines. Last time, the medicine made me feel flu-ish and achy all over for a few days, so I'm dreading feeling crappy on Friday and Saturday, but (hope springs eternal) maybe it won't have those side effects this time.

Typically, I can chase away fear with hope, but right now it's difficult. When I was a teenager, I suffered what now would be probably diagnosed as anxiety and depression but then was considered typical teen angst. One of my recurring nightmares was being sentenced to death and on death row. My crime was never revealed in my dream; I was just awaiting my execution. I'm sure the dream had more to do with feeling a lack of control over my life, which is the very definition of childhood—someone else is forever deciding what you'll do and when you'll do it. It's probably also related to fear of mortality. After all, none of us will get out of here alive. But who wants to admit it? It feels like my new reality is living inside this old nightmare. No control and waiting for the end of life.

Luckily, the past week has provided some wonderful distractions. I enjoyed wrapping gifts and little party favors for Jackson's birthday fete. Another evening, Vivian and I stayed up late wrapping more gifts and laughing like old biddies. My time with Vivian these days is so wonderful; she seems so grown up and poised. Yesterday, I took her to an audition for a radio spot. This child nagged me for nearly a full year to get her an agent, so I finally did. I called an agent, and after a brief audition, they agreed to represent her—two auditions so far. She's been performing in local plays for two years now. I'm so happy Vivian is ambitious; it gives me hope that she'll have a good life filled with satisfying work.

Jackson's birthday celebrations were so fun. Rolls and fruit with family on Saturday morning, dinner at Jack's favorite restaurant on Saturday night, and his kid party on Sunday. The celebration continued on Monday night because we received last-minute Twins tickets from the Angel Foundation. We only stayed until the fifth inning, because early to bed is how we roll.

Each day, my radiation burns appear a little better. My neighbor gave me some aloe vera leaves to keep in the fridge, and that cool aloe gel feels so soothing on my skin. The pain in my hip that led to the discovery of the metastasis is completely gone, but I still walk with a cane for stability. My digestion is much better, and that's improved my quality of life considerably.

Every day, my energy levels improve dramatically. I'm showering each day—yay for me—and I've been out in public quite a bit. Still sleeping nine to ten hours at night, one to three hours during the day, and then I have about two to five hours per day that I'm up and about doing things. The rest of the time I'm resting like a little kitty, often with our big white kitty, Cedric. He lets me spoon him, and he'll purr loudly enough that he helps me rest. Our little Siamese, Shu Shu, is pretty hyper. He'll let us hold him like a baby but won't tolerate snuggling in bed. Our old, old dog, Savannah, sits on the floor next to the bed and pants her stinky dog breath all over the place. She'd be happy to spoon, but she's too smelly for that. Poor girl.

Food couldn't be any less interesting to me these days. I'm forcing down water, juice, and tea to avoid dehydration and eating a few comfort foods here and there. It's amazing how little food it takes to sustain me when I'm not moving my body. One of the medications' side effects is lack of appetite, but I don't think I've lost any weight because I don't need many calories for my daily (in)activities.

Sleep In for a Cure
Saturday, May 12, 2012, 8:23 p.m.

What a difference a day makes. Wednesday I was stressing about my doctor appointment, and by Thursday evening, I felt as if I could conquer the world. Before the end of my bone-medicine infusion, Dr. Anderson told me my tumor markers were back down to the normal range! Typically, it takes a day to get the results, but he's so charming, he must have worked his wiles on the lab to speed up the result. As it turns out, he was expecting the levels to be down because of the radiation. In three weeks, I'll have a PET/CT scan that will give him a better idea of how the Afinitor chemotherapy is working.

Tomorrow for Mother's Day, I'm going to sleep in—but Vivian, my ambitious little eleven-year-old, will be getting up at 5:45 a.m. to do the Race for a Cure. It's a three-mile walk, and while I'd never have the energy for it, I'm very happy she'll be doing the walking in my honor. Friends and family have already donated several hundred dollars to the cause, and Vivian has convinced her Girl Scout troop to walk with her. She loves to raise funds for Susan G. Komen for the Cure. It gives her a positive way to help others facing cancer.

Meanwhile, back at the ranch, I'll sleep in and hopefully get breakfast in bed from my boys. Once Vivian gets home, the boys will go to a Twins game. At some point, I'll have time to myself. I hope to sit out by our pond and read from an amazing little book I found when I was sorting through my mom's things. It's called *Mom, Share Your Life with Me*, and it has 365 questions with room to write. My mom wrote in the book in

2000, and I'm about one-third of the way reading through it. I'm hearing her voice as I read. Some of the stories are things I already know; some are new to me. She was such a sweet woman. I'm getting much comfort from reading this little book she wrote in.

A New Day
Monday, May 21, 2012, 9:46 a.m.

I've had three nights of just four hours of sleep, so proceed with caution.

It's time to start staging our house and looking for a new one. It's yucky to feel like now we're committed to moving. It just doesn't seem fair that getting sick means having to move. So much stress when we don't need it.

Last night, we had dinner with neighbors and stopped to chat with three other neighborhood families on the way home. It's the neighbors, not the house, we'll miss. My secret hope is that the minute we sell our house, we'll find a one-story house within a few blocks so we can have our cake and eat it too.

We know that our financial situation is our own doing. When we were planning our educations and careers, we always said we didn't care about money. We thought making a lot of money meant having fancy cars and nice clothes, which we never cared about. So we devoted our lives to art, nonprofits, and our kids, thinking we were doing the right thing. We thought that an addition to our house for my mom to move in was a great idea; then it didn't pan out because she died too soon, and we were stuck with a supersized mortgage. We thought we were doing the right thing when we didn't actually know the rules. Financial planners say you need six to twelve months of savings, but really, you need six to twelve years of savings, because getting sick is so expensive—even with good health insurance. I don't want to ruin your sense of safety, but this is my truth.

Tomorrow, we'll meet with a financial planner, and maybe he'll see something in our situation that we can't see. Perhaps he'll make a case for us to stay in our house. If so, I'll ask for a second opinion. If two or three people can tell us we can afford to stay in our house *and* take two or three vacations a year, maybe I'll believe it.

I've started a new fitness regimen to get my sleep on a schedule. I'm doing old-school exercises—arm circles, knee bends—think group exercise in Communist China, circa 1950. Typically, I do these exercises outside in the sun and pray nobody is watching me.

Prison Camp
Monday, June 4, 2012, 8:19 p.m.

Yesterday, I cried all through church. From the time I arrived until I left, even walking up to Communion. For a full hour. Part of it was that I didn't get to sleep until 3:00 a.m. I was up late looking for houses in our price range and pulling crime maps of the areas we're considering. In addition to the lack of sleep, the grieving process was top of mind. It feels as if this postcard from Camp Chemo is sent to you from prison camp: I'm here by force, and I have no hope of escape. It feels this way because of the things I've lost with this diagnosis:

My neighborhood—If we move, thanks to the cancer, it isn't the house we'll miss but our backyard, front yard, and neighbors. The other night, a bunch of neighborhood kids and grown-ups congregated in the backyard, and it was so fun. On my best days, I know a smaller house and smaller mortgage will be good for my health, and we'll get to know a bunch of new friends on our new block. On my worst days, I can't even fathom all we need to do to list the house. Plus, I still don't totally understand how it works to sell a house and then find a new one before needing to get out of the old house. Seems like it takes a tremendous amount of faith!

My work—I'm bitterly disappointed that I'm not back to work yet. I really thought I'd be back already, but I need to sleep during the day, and my brain still isn't up to par. Hopefully after meeting with my doctor tomorrow and the financial planner again, I can make some decisions. I want all the clients I've worked with over the years to be taken care of either by me or someone else.

My mobility—Yesterday was our town celebration, complete with parade, bands, kid jumpy inflatables, and fried food. It spans about two miles of one street, open for pedestrians all day. Wade hates crowds, so I usually take the kids or talk Wade into attending. But yesterday, he took the kids. There was no way I could walk even two blocks of the event, let alone two miles.

My ability to care for others—as a mom, this might be the most painful loss. When I was a teen, I started to volunteer at my church and ironically the American Cancer Society. When the opportunity arose, I refused to join the musicians' union because they wouldn't allow volunteering, and I felt it was important to play at least two free harp gigs per year at nursing homes. As a college student, I started to give money (never a full tithe, mind you) to church, public radio, and other organizations because, again, I've always felt it's important to give back when I've been given so much. My whole life, I've had big plans for helping others, and now I'm in no shape to do that. I hope that by giving others an opportunity to help our family, it's a blessing to them too. Everyone's generosity continues to flow, and we appreciate it so much.

Today, Wade and I met with our new priest. That's what happens when you cry through the entire service. I told him I feel like I'm not attending to my spiritual life, because I'm so busy attending to the practical matters of getting our lives organized in the event of my long-term disability or death. He explained that we often compartmentalize our spiritual life and think that we need to be praying or in church to be doing spiritual work. He went on to explain that practical actions can be spiritual in nature. As I'm working on spreadsheets, I'm taking care of my family, and my children are a legacy, so caring for them counts as spiritual practice. His words reminded me of one of my favorite books of all time, *Franny and Zooey* by J. D. Salinger. Franny, a teen drama queen, becomes obsessed with how to "pray ceaselessly"; today, I realized everyday actions can be a form of prayer, praise, thanksgiving, and servitude to God.

It's time to rest and care for my right arm. The lymphedema is a daily struggle, and while I love the warm weather, my arm hates it. So it's time to massage and bandage the old girl so she doesn't swell to the size of Popeye's arm.

Meow! Meow!

Tuesday, June 5, 2012, 8:58 p.m.

My report card arrived today. I received a perfect 4.0! Straight As. That's the way I feel, anyway. It was a wonderful day!

Check out some of my best test scores, from the report now taped up next to my bed. (They're like golf scores—we want low numbers.)

T3 vertebral body 2.1—previously 7.4

Right iliac bone 4.0—previously 8.2

Proximal left femur intertrochanteric 1.9—previously 3.9

L2 vertebral body 2.6—previously 6.5

Inferior anterior left iliac bone 3.4—previously 7.3

And the kicker: "No areas of increased metabolic activity and no new lesions identified." The cancer hasn't spread! The cancer that is there is slowing down with less metabolic activity! Your prayers are working—please keep them up!

This is the first good news we've received in months. I was so excited to see the numbers that I started to meow in the doctor's office. I've been known to break out in meows (or purring) when happy—and hissing when mad. My giddiness continued to amuse my husband, doctor, and nurse through the appointment. Dr. Anderson didn't like the look of my mouth sores, which don't even hurt now. The mouth sores, combined with my fantastic progress, led him to lower the dose of the oral chemo to relieve the side effects. That means a two-day chemo vacation while I wait for the new dose to arrive by mail from the specialty pharmacy.

I'll get a blood draw next week (can't remember why). Then one month later, I'll see Dr. Anderson for a blood draw and bone juice. Then a PET scan a few months later. We still have things to accomplish, but for now it's all good news!

When I asked about my energy levels and work, he said to give it another month or two. That was disappointing, because today I felt like I could conquer the world.

We celebrated by using some cash a fellow survivor sent for a meal out, and we toasted to my dear Dr. Anderson.

5:00 P.M. Wake-Up Call

Saturday, June 9, 2012, 3:40 a.m.

It's official: I'm nocturnal. Yesterday, I woke up around 1:00 p.m., and today I woke up at 5:00 p.m. Ugh.

The culprit for my lack of energy is the Aredia, a.k.a. "bone juice," I received on Tuesday. It's left me with terrible flu-like symptoms, nausea, and a record number of mouth sores—seven. Everything I eat and drink, including water, hurts.

Tomorrow, I'll get a new bottle of the magic lidocaine swish to help dull the mouth pain. On Monday, I'll call my dentist to get fitted for another mouth splint. I've been grinding my teeth so much at night there are sharp edges and cracks in the splint I bought years ago. The splints aren't covered by insurance (yet fixing cracked or broken teeth is covered—go figure), so it will be a big indulgence. The last one cost over $400, but it will be worth it to make my mouth and jaw more comfortable.

Hopefully, my next dose of Aredia will have fewer side effects. Unlike traditional chemo, which has a cumulative effect, the Afinitor pills have the most intense side effects in the first few doses. Dr. Anderson promised fewer side effects next month. In the meantime, I have to watch for fever, because infections can start in the mouth and spread into the blood system. So far, no fever. Normally, it takes about three weeks for the mouth sores I've had in the past to heal. I hope these will heal faster.

Speaking of hope, one of the very first gifts I received after this metastatic breast cancer diagnosis was a book, *When Everything Falls Apart* by a Buddhist nun named Pema Chödrön. She explains that both hope and fear are problematic because they keep us from living in the moment. She also writes that seeking security leads to suffering. That is at the core of my suffering right now. I've worked so hard to provide security for myself and my family, but it's an impossible goal. Two different sermons I heard years ago have been bouncing around in my brain, both centered around the idea that there is no security except in God. In practice, though, it's difficult to make friends with the groundlessness beneath our feet. Sigh. This experience is forcing me to live without making plans for the future; and yet being responsible with our resources is critical to making them last as long as possible. There must be some wisdom in this pair of opposites.

It's difficult to watch Wade working so hard to get our house in order to possibly sell it for a more affordable home. I wish he could have a break from it all. I know from the experience of caring for my mother that it's much easier to be the sick one than to be the caregiver. Please include Wade in your prayers. I feel bad for him because once upon a time, he was a teenager who wanted to marry a pretty girl, and now he's stuck with an old woman who, to quote Jackson, "just sleeps all the time and never gets out of bed."

OK, I'm going to try to abandon hope in the Buddhist sense, not the Dante sense, and live in this moment. I'm going to enjoy a climate-controlled house (thanks to the air conditioner Wade installed today); the memory of a beautiful night with an outdoor fire by the pond with the kids; a nice evening walk when I smelled seven varieties of roses, some sweet, some spice—all wonderful. And the memory of yesterday, finding the very first ripe raspberry in our alley garden. So much beauty all around, and I don't want to waste it on worry.

Mother's Day

Sunday, June 17, 2012, 10:59 p.m.

Yes, I know today is Father's Day. We celebrated with a picnic in the park and gifts for Wade. Vivian and I gave him a Buddha head for the pond, along with some aquatic plants our fish desperately need for cover. Jackson gave him a less tranquil treat, an afternoon at the movies to see *The Avengers*.

The reason this postcard from Camp Chemo is titled "Mother's Day" is because everyone has been asleep already for over an hour, and I've had time for something amazing to sink in. It makes me feel like I'm the one who received a precious gift today. In fact, tears started to stream down my face. Here's what happened . . .

The last few days, Vivian has been asking how much money she has in the bank. She's talking about something she wants to save for, but she can't tell us what it is.

Here's the backstory: Before the cancer metastasized, we'd been saving for a new kitchen. The current layout is impossible. The cabinets are from the 1920s, and each time something broke, we'd say we should just redo the whole thing—but I refused to go into debt for it. Anyway—our dishwasher broke on Friday. Wade located the broken part online, but it will take a few days to arrive. Vivian has been doing dishes like a little trooper, and today she asked how much a new kitchen costs. We told her an approximate amount. Vivian knows that after my diagnosis, we put any home improvements on hold in favor of seeking less expensive housing and more cash in the bank for future medical expenses.

Here's what sent tears streaming down my face tonight: As Vivian was going to sleep tonight, she confided that she wanted to save up enough money to get me a new kitchen. But when she learned the price, she realized there's no way she'd be able to save that much. I told her that it doesn't matter if she had the money or not; it's gift enough that she would even think of it. Tears are streaming down my cheeks again as I think about the amazingly generous little soul sleeping upstairs. I often remind her she gets that generosity from her grandma.

A thunderstorm is brewing with all the rolling noise and flashes of light, so now it's time for me to rest and enjoy Mother Nature's show.

Survivor's Guilt

Tuesday, June 19, 2012, 9:18 p.m.

The last few days, I've been experiencing survivor's guilt.

On Sunday, as I blithely wrote about raspberries and the beautiful storm brewing, a dearly loved friend was passing away. My mother's best friend in her last twenty years, or maybe even thirty, was a sweet and sturdy woman named Aiko. Like my mother, Aiko worked her entire career in public health fighting as a champion for the health of children in Minnesota and across the nation. My mother's blood sister passed away in the 1990s, and soon after, I started hearing her and Aiko talk about each other as "sisters." They even looked like twins, the same height, weight, permed (and I mean this lovingly) old-lady hair, and the same glasses. Even their gait was similar. The only noticeable difference was that Mom was of Swedish heritage, and Aiko was of Japanese heritage. Quick to laugh, Aiko also was about as polite and formal as they come. She would walk arm in arm with my mom the way women of their generation would do so sweetly. She was generous, often thinking of our family. Despite spending World War II unlawfully detained in a Japanese internment camp, she wasn't bitter—quite the opposite. She was an amazing gardener, with a huge raspberry patch and massive zucchini that my mom would make into delicious bread every summer. During zucchini bread season, that's all I'd eat for a week, a thick slab of butter on each slice. Yum. When I called Aiko to tell her my mother had died, she was shocked. She said, "It should have been me. I should have gone first." Aiko's survivor's guilt was because she'd had heart trouble for many years. And yet my mom preceded her in death.

Yesterday, Wade came into the room and told me, "Your cousin called to say Aiko died 'in the storm last night,' and your mom has a best friend in heaven now." I felt so sad and guilty. I had savored that storm, feeling cozy in my home while the world was losing a dear soul. The only consolation is imagining them in heaven, walking arm in arm to get their hair permed and making each other laugh all the way.

The Man in the Mirror
Friday, June 22, 2012, 2:36 a.m.

This title could be a Michael Jackson reference. (I love that song.) But it's more literal. I look more and more like a man all the time.

My cancer feeds on estrogen, so job one was to remove as much estrogen as possible—namely, the ovaries. I ditched them back in 2008. Menopause had started a few months earlier with my first round of chemo. Then for years, I took tamoxifen, which blocks estrogen. But I can't completely escape estrogen. Some is made in the pituitary gland, and some hangs out in fat cells. So now I'm on another estrogen-blocking drug, exemestane. On top of that, my daily Afinitor chemo pill creates side effects, including acne and weak fingernails and toenails. Look closely and you'll see my facial hair has become darker and more prolific. Wade and I noticed it on the same day. We joked about starting an old-school freak show featuring me as the bearded lady.

It's getting more difficult to fight all the manly attributes I see in the mirror. For years, my figure was a consistent 34-23-34. That changed with kids, chemo-induced menopause, and this new regimen has me even more barrel-chested and waistless. Now, I can only wear women's clothing if it has full elastic at the waist, because my hips and waist are only a couple of inches apart. A manlier figure.

In positive beauty news, my hair is growing—halfway down my back, just how I like it—but it's getting whiter and whiter all the time. Once it's 100 percent white, I'll stop coloring it, but for now, I like having the long, dark hair of my youth. It's a way to feel more girly.

Amazingly, my wonderful hubby still sees the best in me, whiskers and all. A testament to his commitment and love.

Step One

Tuesday, July 10, 2012, 10:28 p.m.

Each day, I have thoughts I want to share by writing—but instead, I most-ly sleep during the day and then try (unsuccessfully) to sleep at night. It's really awful. Got some new sleep medication—I'm so out of shape that when I try to lie down to sleep, I toss and turn, and my legs literally jump when I'm in the bed, as if they wanted more exercise during the day, but I can't manage more than two or three blocks of walking per day.

This sucks.

It's like step one in the twelve-step program: "I am powerless over my disease, and my life has become unmanageable." I've been trying to man-age my life for the last three and a half months, and I'm failing miserably.

My income—meaning my ability to work or not work—is being reviewed by the disability insurance company now. My doctor says I shouldn't work, and I know deep down he's right, but I'm still fighting to keep up at work. Losing my career is perhaps the most painful loss.

My ability to plan for the future hinges on scans and blood work.

My emotional life feels like a disaster.

How could I keep such a great attitude in the past, and now I'm falling apart?

I've been reading various books about Buddhism, and it all leads back to the present moment. The masters teach that there is no ability to plan the future, and the ground under our feet is just an illusion. So what "illusions" do I count on at this moment? I have a nice house (but I'm incredibly worried we'll lose it); I have a comfy bed; my tummy is full; my mouth sores are better (thanks to a visit to the dentist today); my nosebleeds are fewer (thanks to some lotion my nurse told me to put in my nose); and I have a nice sleeping pill waiting for me.

My cancer tumor markers keep going down, which is good. Howev-er, my cholesterol is way up as a medication side effect. It's all too much medication for my body to process.

I can't believe my mantra ever was "Keep Calm and Carry On." I'm a miserable failure; I can't even do cancer correctly. I can't believe I ever cared about facial hair and makeup. It's all so tiny compared with the current mess.

There's so much more I want to write, but I just wanted to check in and ask you to please continue to pray for us.

My MRI with David Sedaris

Thursday, July 12, 2012, 10:53 p.m.

Bottom line, I had a great day. Felt like myself for the first time in ages. My recent brain MRI (to rule out anything physical and nasty going on up there) went fine. I'm feeling so good it seems impossible that anything could be wrong with my brain, but I won't receive the results until next week.

It was my first brain scan, so I wasn't sure what to expect. I've had a breast MRI, so I knew it would be noisy. They put my head on a pillow, placed earplugs in my ears, wedged cushions around my head, and fit a sort of plastic mask over my face. They give you a little button to hold in case you want out of the machine.

Then: knocking, buzzing, clanging, and whirring. Not at any regular intervals. I tried to just relax and imagine lying on a beach, but it's difficult with all that noise. Then, with no warning, I wanted to jump up, but I couldn't because they need me to stay still for the images.

The machine's clattering is loud—lawnmower- or machine gun–level decibels. Even with earplugs. MRIs always leave me feeling shell-shocked, because the sounds remind me of warfare.

The tech checks in, saying, "We're starting the next sequence, eight minutes." So I at least know the noise will endure for eight minutes before it stops. It's very reassuring to hear the tech's voice over the radio. He sits in the next room, and through a big window, he can see the soles of my feet peeking out of the machine.

This time when the buzzing started, I tried to think of a loud noise that felt positive, so I pretended I was on *The Price Is Right* (old-school, with Bob Barker) and I'd just won a prize. The buzz told me I'd won. The studio audience was going wild, and I was jumping up and down. The announcer's voice shouted, "You've won . . . A *NEW* CAR!!!" The curtain rose on a lovely white convertible with buttermilk leather seats. I ran over and jumped in the driver's seat as the crowd continued to applaud. This went on for a while, long enough for the first MRI sequence. I had time to win several convertibles, including a gray Chrysler Sebring, a rust-orange vintage Euro convertible, and a baby-blue Audi, a replica of the one Reese Witherspoon drove in *Legally Blonde*. The Audi also came with a little Chihuahua just like her movie dog, Bruiser.

My biggest problem in the world was where I would park all these amazing cars. The clanging noise continued as I spun the giant wheel and played the Showcase Showdown. I won fabulous vacations and an entirely new wardrobe of clothes, selected just for me by my own personal stylist.

Then the whirring noise started, and it took a while to figure this one out. I've got it—it sounds like a puddle-jumper plane. Suddenly, I was aboard a private jet. All decked out with lovely leather seats set up like sectional couches. Just like the private jets in soap operas. Maybe these well-appointed jets exist in real life? Suddenly, I was flying to the French Riviera with my BFF, David Sedaris.

If you don't know of David Sedaris, think back to young adulthood and try to remember the funniest, smartest, friendliest person you knew—someone with the exact same sense of humor as you. This is the best way to describe David Sedaris, an American humorist, called by some "the Rock Star of Writers." I love all his books, but my favorite has to be *Me Talk Pretty One Day*.

Soon David and I were driving along a beautiful, two-lane, curvy freeway in a white Mercedes convertible. We were laughing and joking about what makes for better stories: growing up with five wacky siblings (David) or as an only lonely (me). We laughed as we tried to speak French despite our limited vocabularies.

When the car ran out of gas, we just chuckled and decided to buy a new one. We settled on a cobalt-blue Mercedes convertible and drove it straight to the beach. We got out and ran along the cool grass to the warm sand. David was surprisingly buff in his swim trunks (he'd *never* wear a

Speedo, not even in France), and we were the most beautiful and famous people on the beach. Even though we were famous, nobody bothered us, because our fans are the respectful types; they're just happy to gaze at us from afar.

The MRI's clanging started. I realized it was like a sound a casino slot machine would make. David and I suddenly appeared in a glamorous Monaco casino. We didn't gamble—we never would because it's immoral—but as we walked through the casino to see a stage show, I absentmindedly pulled the lever of a machine, and gold coins start pouring out. We laughed and filled bucket after bucket with the coins. A bunch of my girlfriends showed up with buckets, and we all laughed as the coins poured out for "three and a half minutes," as Joe, the MRI tech, told me at the start of this sequence. David and I found it hilarious to win so much money, because we were already so rich.

When the whirring started again, we were back on the private jet—after donating our Mercedes convertibles to charity, of course. Once the knocking and clanging started, we were in Hawaii, at a luau, with the sea, fire, dancers, drummers, music, and a feast. It was night and day at the same time, with a brilliant sun.

Before long, more whirring, and we were back on the jet, headed to South Beach. We hadn't needed a car in Hawaii, but we decided a 1950s vintage, pastel-peach Cadillac would complement Miami's art deco buildings.

In Miami, we didn't even need to buy the car ourselves; the hotel concierge bought it for us, based on our exact order. Each car we'd had so far came with the glove box filled with Grace Kelly–style scarves so my hair wouldn't tangle in the wind, and the center consoles were each filled with designer sunglasses. David told me I looked fabulous in each pair. When we returned to the hotel, we learned that my personal stylist had sent me a brand-new, Miami-appropriate wardrobe. I was tickled pink. Again, David insisted I looked beautiful in all the outfits, and we spent hours enjoying the South Beach nightlife and telling side-splitting stories. This is the land of beautiful people, but we were once again the most beautiful and famous.

The MRI tech's voice interrupted, "Last sequence, four minutes."

David and I continued to dance, dine, try on clothes, and drive around. We ditched the vintage Caddie for a brand-new, vintage-styled white Thunderbird with a red interior, and a faux-wood dash panel and steering wheel.

Soon it was time to say good-bye. Wade and the kids missed me, and David's partner, Hugh, missed him. We were happy to have such nice people waiting for us at home. We donated the Caddy and T-bird to charity, hugged our good-byes, and promised to meet up in Sedona at a fabulous spa we'd always wanted to visit together.

Finished with the MRI, I changed back into my street clothes, and as I stepped into my old tan Subaru station wagon, I felt rich and lucky, as if I'd really just returned from a fabulous vacation.

Back at home, Wade laughed when I told him about my MRI with David Sedaris. I apologized that I didn't take Wade with me instead. Wade admitted that a gay man would probably be much more interested in my outfits, convertibles, and matching sunglasses than he would have been.

It was so nice David could come with me today.

Workweek Weekend

Saturday, July 28, 2012, 10:05 p.m.

Health update—my brain MRI showed no cancer, and my brain is normal! (Hold the jokes, please!) This is such a big relief.

This week, I went back to work with a reduced schedule, doing a small portion of my regular duties. On Monday, I figured I'd do everything just like before . . . but by Wednesday, I felt my stamina slip. It's bitterly disappointing to have such crippling fatigue. Each day I'd get home around two and then sleep for a few hours. My brain wants to do everything I used to do, but my energy level just isn't the same. It was still gratifying to be back with people I love to see every day, in a place I respect, doing work that makes me feel competent. Next week, I'll work Monday through Wednesday. Then I'll meet with my bosses and HR to figure out how to go forward.

Two pieces of great financial news arrived this week. First, I realized I'd misunderstood my company life insurance deal. I'd thought it would go away after my health insurance COBRA period ends. As it turns out, the life insurance will remain intact. I can't explain my relief. Some people may think it's weird to be excited about money my family will receive after I die, but it lets me breathe easier to know Wade and the kids will have help to get back on their feet after I'm gone. This news doesn't mean we're going to be rich (we never set out to be), but the odds of us (or them) ending up in the poorhouse have decreased.

The other good news is that it's very unlikely I can be denied payments by my disability insurance company. That's been my biggest fear. On top of that, no matter what the disability insurance company tries to do with my claim, I'm guaranteed Social Security—which is too little to live on, but it's still better than nothing. Turns out the US government has something called Compassionate Allowances. I love that our government has anything with the word *compassionate* in it—that gives me hope for the future. The Compassionate Allowances are a list of 165 diseases that automatically permit Social Security payments. I looked down the list, which begins with Acute Leukemia and ends with Zellweger Syndrome, and whoo-hoo! There's my disease: "Breast Cancer—with distant metastases or inoperable or unresectable." It's so odd to be happy that it's inoperable. You should check out this list of diseases. There are so many I've not heard of that I want to learn about: Angelman Syndrome, Batten Disease, Cri du Chat Syndrome, Stiff Person Syndrome, and Tricuspid Atresia. They all sound way worse and more fascinating than cancer, right?

Last night, we had friends over for dinner. Jackson had a blast with their three little boys. Activities included spontaneous wrestling, a push-up contest, digging for worms in the mud, feeding worms to the fish in our pond, a bonfire, and a truly epic light saber bout. Vivian had a friend sleeping over, and they helped keep watch over all those boys.

Are You There, HIPAA? It's Me, Camille.

Wednesday, August 1, 2012, 8:06 p.m.

Tomorrow, I'll see my oncologist. My last visit was slightly traumatic for two reasons.

First, I encountered a very sweet church friend and her husband in the waiting room. It's never a good sign to see someone you know at the oncology office. It felt so terrible to hear she had cancer, and I said all the things I hate to hear when I tell people my news: "Oh no," "I'm so sorry this happened to you," "Chemo sucks," "This is awful." I later said I'm sorry I reacted this way. She was gracious, but I still felt guilty.

After my appointment, I went to the infusion room, which has chairs about two or three feet away from each other. I took a spot next to a man and the two women sitting with him. I closed my eyes to rest while my bone juice infused. Through the thin curtain that separated us, I could hear the man protesting as his wife said, "Just take the last few sips of soup." I thought, *Leave the poor man alone. He doesn't feel well.* I know what it's like to be so sick that you don't want to eat or drink anything at all.

The nurse was in and out, and based on the comments she made, I knew the man was getting IV fluid for dehydration. His wife left to seek more soup, and I heard his grown daughter inquire about his will. She was talking about the best way to set it up because something in the tax code changed from $3 million to $5 million—and she didn't want him to have to pay any more tax than was required. I remember thinking it odd to sit next to a guy with millions (and a daughter who seemed anxious to get her hands on it) while I was fretting about getting back to work and my disability insurance. Soon the wife returned with more soup. (Geez, leave the poor man alone. He's getting IV fluids; he doesn't need the soup.) Then I heard Dr. Anderson's distinctive voice: "Last time, your number was 1523; this time, it's 3045. I've never seen them increase so quickly. I'm surprised."

Before I had time to try to figure out which number he was talking about, Dr. Anderson said, "I'm sorry to tell you, there's nothing more I can do for you."

Oh wow.

"I can give you a referral to Mayo or the university hospital, but I don't think there's anything they'll be able to do, either."

"How long does he have?" one of the women asked.

"Two or three weeks." Dr. Anderson went on to tell the man not to check into a hospital. "There's nothing they can do for you," he said. Instead, he advised getting set up with hospice. After a bit more discussion about IV fluids and transfusions, Dr. Anderson, "I'll see you tomorrow for the transfusion."

"What if I don't come in tomorrow?" the man asked.

"You won't make it through the weekend." This was a Thursday.

Dr. Anderson left. Through the curtain, I heard the man say, "I've lived a good life." He cried with his family a little bit, and his wife scurried off to get yet more soup.

The daughter continued on her same track, "So, Dad, who's your estate attorney? We really need to get that taken care of right away."

I wanted to jump through the curtain, shake her, and say, "Leave the poor (rich) guy alone! The money doesn't mean a thing!"

To be fair, maybe the family has a charity they support, and the daughter wanted to preserve the wealth for that legacy. Maybe she wanted to keep a financial mess from absorbing her mom's life. Or maybe she was just greedy. Whatever the context, I felt her timing was awful, and she should have waited a day—even an hour—before getting back to the business of the will. Everyone deals with grief and death in their own way, so I'm trying not to judge but finding it very difficult.

I told this story to a group of friends, and they had a different take on the conversation. They were like, "Holy HIPAA violation, Batman!" HIPAA, the Health Insurance Portability and Accountability Act, should protect health-care privacy. Nobody said the man's name, so I still have no idea who he was, and his health information didn't mean much to me, but still—where's HIPAA when you need it?

Driving home from my infusion that day, I couldn't help but cry. I'd been sitting there worrying myself sick about money, all the while sitting alongside someone who clearly had more than enough money for himself, his family, and even me. But all that money can't buy him another minute of time or a family who'll let him decide whether or not to drink the damn soup. Would he trade some of his money for a few of my spare weeks?

Today, make sure *you* decide if you want the soup or not. Live in peace and let others live or die in peace, whatever their choice. Keep calm and carry on.

Trauma-Free
Friday, August 3, 2012, 5:19 p.m.

Yesterday's doctor appointment was trauma-free, thank goodness. My white count and platelets are low, which means my ability to fight infections is compromised, and my blood won't clot as easily as it should. The levels aren't so low as to be critically dangerous, but Dr. Anderson will lower the Afinitor dose. Afinitor was finally FDA approved last week, so hopefully more people will go on it and we'll learn more about side effects and the results of its long-term use.

Birthday Bliss
Sunday, August 5, 2012, 9:50 p.m.

Today was my birthday, and the day went exactly as I'd planned.

I attended the church picnic with my family. A parishioner was baptized in the Mississippi River. It's the first river baptism I've seen—pretty amazing.

I forced my family to do a jigsaw puzzle with me. I love puzzles, but nobody in my house loves them quite as much as I do (hence the forcing).

We went to a dog-friendly event along the big retail street in town. We brought our sweet Savannah and saw many cute dogs.

Sunday dinner at Melissa and Uri's house, complete with gifts and a massive carrot cake.

Thanks for all the well wishes. Having a birthday to celebrate makes me very happy!

Update
Friday, September 28, 2012, 2:11 p.m.

My health update couldn't be better. The most recent PET/CT scan showed no evidence of disease! It doesn't mean the cancer is gone, just that it's so inactive the numbers were too small to record. I should be jumping up and down at the news, but Afinitor causes severe fatigue. I'll take a good scan over a bad one any day—but the rest of my body tells me this fatigue isn't over, not by a long shot.

Mouth sores are another lingering side effect of the Afinitor. I've adjusted by avoiding abrasive foods (chips, toast, breakfast cereal) and always drinking out of straws to avoid further aggravating the mouth sores. It's also driving my bad cholesterol through the roof, and it makes my good cholesterol low. My triglycerides and blood sugar are high. This means I have to eat very carefully, avoiding fat and carbs. Loads of fruits and veggies and small portions of everything else will hopefully help me avoid a heart attack and diabetes. I'll be so mad if I have a heart attack! I'm determined to not die from cancer, but if anything else gets me, I'll be pissed! Ha!

My career as I've known it for fifteen-plus years has ended. It was very sad to go on long-term disability, but it's the only way to cope with this cancer. The mild cognitive impairment from the chemo has left my brain unable to handle the intellectual demands of my work. The physical energy required for work is no longer available to me. Afternoon naps are frowned upon at most workplaces. My ability to process and handle everyday stress allows me only minimal activities. I'm still holding out hope for a complete metastatic breast cancer cure. I'd gladly trade in cancer for the stress that comes along with earning a living. But realistically, the best way to attend to my health is to stay home and focus on rest and following doctors' orders.

Wade noted that I've recently come out of mourning. I've been mourning my job, my livelihood, and my concept of myself as a competent person and a working mother. I'm starting to accept that work is behind me and that staying home to attend to my health is the right thing to do. Wade and I have switched roles: he's working the hours I used to work, and I'm taking care of the house and the kids. Now I'm helping kids with homework after school like he used to do. Still, I can't even do as much around the house as I used to do between 9:00 p.m. and midnight before cancer, when I was working full-time.

Thanks to tons of physical therapy, I've been able to finally ditch my cane. I can even walk through Target! No more motorized store carts for me. I'll miss crashing them into store displays, but giving them up is a good thing. While I can't walk all I want (no state fair for me this year), it feels great to walk more than one city block without disabling pain. I've also moved back upstairs to my own bedroom! One flight of stairs is hardly a problem, most of the time. All these things are worth celebrating.

My very first Social Security check will arrive in November. I'm terrified when I think about the tiny fraction of my former pay it represents. I think about how this is a fixed income and I'll never, ever get a raise beyond a small annual cost-of-living adjustment. Age forty to fifty are sometimes described as the "prime earning years," and I feel cheated to be missing out on mine. I look at my retirement statements, realizing I can no longer afford to add to those accounts. It's enough to make me worry about growing old, even as the odds of growing old shrink.

Good-Bye, Savannah

Sunday, September 30, 2012, 8:11 p.m.

Today, we said a difficult good-bye to our dear dog, Savannah. She's been declining over the last few months. With the help of our vet, we decided she was suffering too much. She couldn't walk up the front steps or play, and she wasn't eating much.

We sat with Savannah all afternoon outside near the pond. We hugged her, and Vivian tied a special ribbon around her neck. Her black fur shone in the sun. Such a beautiful dog. We admired her beautiful eyelashes and pretty face one last time. A vet came to the house, and we all gathered around Savannah to say good-bye. We said prayers from *The Book of Common Prayer* and cried when she was gone. It was a peaceful passing, but we'll miss her very much. Wade wrapped her in cloth and lowered her into her final resting spot, and we threw flowers in as I read more prayers. I couldn't find my modern prayer book, so we read from the one that says, "Earth to earth, ashes to ashes, dust to dust." We spent a lot of time talking about sadness, loss, and grief.

Wade and I found Savannah at the local humane society when I was pregnant with Vivian. Savannah was two and a half, and "half black Lab, half Doberman," according to her paperwork. She had lived with kids and other pets. The reason for surrender was because her owner had died. It was so sad to imagine kids losing a parent and their dog at the same time. Savannah knew her name, so we kept it for her. She was well trained and could sit and stay and walk on a leash with no problems. We could tell she'd been well loved by her first family. Vivian's very first word was "dog," and before she could say "Savannah," she would say "See-AHH-dun," which became my favorite nickname for the first dog I ever loved.

I have so many favorite memories of her—Vivian dressing her up, both kids laying their heads on her, my mom kicking the ball to her end-lessly in the backyard. A favorite memory happened just a few weeks ago. Vivian was at a friend's house, and she scammed her way into a sleepover. I gathered her things for the overnight stay and let Savannah ride along as I delivered them. She loved the car and would sit in the front seat with a big, open-mouthed smile on her doggy face. We drove to deliver Vivian's sleepover items with the car windows down on that beautiful fall night. We were two old gals out for a little joy ride. That was the last happy car trip we took together, and it will always be a special memory.

I'd resisted putting her down, even though Wade knew it was the right thing. The decision hits a little too close to home.

New Love

Sunday, October 14, 2012, 2:55 p.m.

My last oncologist visit was good. My cholesterol and triglycerides are back in the normal range, so getting strict with my diet in combination with a new cholesterol medication worked. The tumor markers are holding steady. In the weeks leading up to the visit, I was worried that cholesterol and triglycerides were clogging my heart with gunk. I began to feel something in my chest that I thought must be a heart attack. When I asked my doctor if I'm heading to heart trouble, he said, "I'll worry about your heart. You're doing well. Your tumors are shrinking. You're in a golden age. You'll have things to worry about in the future—but for now, there's nothing to worry about."

His reassurances reminded me of a passage from Matthew that comforted my mom when she was dying: "Don't borrow worry, because worry will find you in the future."

These days, I hear good news with a different ear. I know now that everything good is temporary. I'm glad to have recently joined a support group for people with metastatic breast cancer. We're able to articulate things like this to each other, say things and hear things that aren't spoken outside the support group. This feeling that "good is temporary, so don't get too excited" is what we discussed last week in group. It's just a part of reality. One of my fellow group members said that since her last good doctor's appointment, she's felt she's living on a "cusp of grace." That's the perfect description of where I'm at right now.

Our family was so sad to have lost our beautiful Savannah. Since my diagnosis, we've been looking to add a Chihuahua to our animal family. Wade and the kids gave me a book about these darling little creatures for Mother's Day, and Vivian contributed more than ninety dollars to the Chihuahua cause. Her generosity seems endless. Wade was really sad in the days after Savannah died and looked on the humane society website for a Chihuahua. Four babies and a mom were on the site—which is surprising, because they rarely get Chihuahuas. The next morning, they were all adopted. Vivian hit "refresh" that afternoon, and one of them was back on the site. We all jumped in the car and drove just over the speed limit to the humane society. And so . . . introducing Lupita Maria Rosalita Shivers Quivers. Lupie, or Lulu, for short. (It was either that or Eleanor Roosevelt. A little dog needs a big name.)

Lupie has brought new life into our house and backyard. She runs and jumps and is so cute. I often squeak at the top of my voice and spontaneously compose songs for her. She is only two pounds and will probably grow to about six pounds. Poor little thing was found with her mom, her siblings, and a few other Chihuahuas under a trailer at a trailer park. She is literally trailer trash. Our love for her proves that one person's trash really is another person's treasure.

Now my support group is up to 30 percent of us having new puppies and 25 percent new convertibles. This spring I hope to join the convertible group too. Funny how a terminal diagnosis makes people want puppies and convertibles.

The new love we've found with Lupie reminds me of hymn number 204 from the Episcopal Church's *The Hymnal 1982*:

Now the green blade riseth from the buried grain,
Wheat that in dark earth many days has lain;
Love lives again, that with the dead has been:
Love is come again, like wheat that springeth green.

When our hearts are wintry, grieving, or in pain,
Thy touch can call us back to life again;
Fields of our hearts that dead and bare have been:
Love is come again. like wheat that springeth green.

The hymn is about Easter, but right now for our family, it's about our own Easter, the resurrection of hope, new life, and new love. And cuteness. Lots and lots of cuteness.

Mutated Cancer

Sunday, November 4, 2012, 9:11 a.m.

Last week, Dr. Anderson explained that my recent scan showed activity on my left hip, a spot that hasn't been active before. That, along with an increased tumor marker, means the cancer probably mutated and has become resistant to the treatment that has been working so well since spring. No one or two tests can tell the whole story, so we need to test again in six weeks. If the tumors appear more active, we'll know the current treatment has stopped working. We can't increase the dose of Afinitor because my white counts and platelets are too low; my body can't handle a higher dose. However, it's possible this activity on the scan could be bone regeneration and nothing to worry about.

As Dr. Anderson described it, we only have so many bullets to use on this cancer. So he can't just discard this treatment until he knows for sure it isn't working. I like the image of pointing the bullets at the cancer, because sometimes with all the side effects, it feels like the bullets are aimed at me instead.

Last weekend, I was a nervous wreck waiting for my Monday PET/CT scan. I was having nightmares—Jackson goes missing, my doctor decides to put me back on the horrible TAC chemo I had years ago, that sort of thing.

The recent news from my doctor had me saying to Wade, "I don't want to die." I want to see what happens to my kids. I want to be here to help them grow.

Scan Results

Friday, December 14, 2012, 8:26 p.m.

First, let me say that I have two happy, healthy, and compassionate kids, so in terms of the important things, life is good.

Yesterday, we learned my PET/CT scan revealed the spot on my left hip from scan six weeks ago has grown. My white counts are even lower than before. These factors, along with the medication side effects, explain my extreme fatigue.

Of course this isn't the news we wanted, but it's not as bad as it could be. Still no cancer in any soft tissue. Dr. Anderson recommended a short course of five radiation treatments for the left hip. We'll stop the daily Afinitor for a few weeks. This will hopefully allow my white counts to increase.

Wade and I saw the news as positive yesterday, because the cancer is still treatable. Today, I'm not feeling so upbeat. Between the added fatigue from yesterday's monthly bone shot and the terrible news of the Sandy Hook school shooting, I've been sleeping most of the day with my little Lupita Maria and eating comfort food. Wade really needs a break, so I hope to be up and running tomorrow and able to take care of the kids so he can get out for a much-needed break.

As you pray for those involved in the Sandy Hook school shooting, please also send some healing prayers my way. Also please pray that Lupita Maria stops peeing on our bed and pooping under the Christmas tree.

Nuclear Christmas

Monday, December 31, 2012, 5:06 p.m.

My mom and I always had Christmas Day with just the two of us when I was growing up. When I got a little older, my grandma would join us. We also had a big Christmas Eve celebration with extended family and friends. So I always wondered what it would be like to have a Christmas with a nuclear family—mom, dad, sister, and brother.

This year, I got my Nuclear Christmas. It was just as wonderful as I'd imagined as a kid. I got to spend a bunch of time in the kitchen baking and cooking with Wade. Watching the kids opening gifts was, of course, the highlight. Church on Christmas Eve was lovely. But I still missed seeing my cousins at their big Christmas Eve party, but they were out of town this year.

This Christmas season, whenever I'd see a Christmas tree at a party, I'd spend a few minutes just looking at it. We had a great time putting up our tree—a "Chinese Pine" fake tree we got after Christmas last year. Our historic tree that was knocked over on a stage by Courtney Love in the 1990s finally had to be discarded a couple of years ago. The cats had peed on it in the basement. (I'm sure it wasn't a comment on her music.) We've had real trees the last couple of years, but our brand-new "Chinese Pine" is much cheaper than a real tree. I piled on the ornaments, and Vivian insisted on tinsel because that's something Mom always had on her tree.

We typically do a year-end gift to charity, and the last few years we've involved the kids in the decision of which organizations to include. This year, Vivian chose the humane society in thanks for Lupie, and Jackson chose the American Cancer Society "so that Mommy can live longer." Hearing him say that was bittersweet. I didn't realize that he connected cancer with early mortality, but I'm glad to know what's on his mind.

On Friday, I saw Dr. Anderson, and he's happy with all my numbers. My white count, platelets, and iron are all low—but they're higher than they were before I started the Afinitor vacation. He wants me to start the Afinitor again on January 10. In the meantime, I'm enjoying almost normal energy levels and eating anything I want, including potato chips, crunchy cinnamon snack toast, and pineapple—all things I had to avoid when the mouth sores were bad.

I've been burning the candle at both ends with my extra energy and just using it up with great abandon. It's really fun to not have to ration my energy for a little while. Jackson has benefited by having more of my attention for his Lego creations. Vivian finally convinced me to start teaching her harp again; we'll see how long I have energy for that.

My support group continues to be a great comfort. However, one of our members, Karen, learned her cancer has spread to her brain. We don't know exactly what it means for her yet. She admitted she'd been thinking of her life in terms of many more years, but now she understands it will be much shorter. Karen is so calm. It's very inspiring. It's also sobering. She'd been feeling really good; her only symptom was a bit of numbness in her face. No big headaches or major issues. We talk a lot in the group about how strange it is that we can't tell what's going on in our own bodies. Sometimes one of us will have a scan that we're thinking will be just fine and then bad news. Or vice versa.

Operation Zero Deductible

Tuesday, January 8, 2013, 6:09 p.m.

I've just knocked on wood to avoid a jinx because I've stayed healthy and uninjured for the first eight days of the New Year. Only forty-three hours until Operation Zero Deductible begins when I get my bone injection. Operation Zero Deductible is a plan to have the bone injection drug company pay my deductible for the year. It's three thousand dollars, so fingers crossed that it will work.

This chemo vacation is so wonderful. I haven't felt this good in a year. So much energy, and I'm using it all up. Much of my time is being spent organizing our house so that when I have less energy, everything will be easier to get done. One of my new year's resolutions is to maximize our home's storage space. The others are:

* Have more fun
* Wear false eyelashes more often
* Be gentle with myself and my family
* Live with the seasons—notice them
   and let them direct my activities

I've even started doing our taxes already. Our appointment with the accountant isn't until next month, but if I have the energy now, may as well get started.

I've also been spending a lot of time feasting—in the literal and religious senses. I've been overindulging in food and fun. Mostly by playing Legos with Jackson, watching TV with Vivian, and snuggling with Lupita Maria (she's on my legs right now). And I've been doing some meditating. When I'm in church, it's so moving to see the crucifer walking down the aisle with the cross. As an Episcopalian, I bow to the cross as it passes, which makes me imagine what it will be like the first time I experience the Lord in heaven; I imagine needing to bow and cover my eyes to the light. It's wonderful to think of a place that is all love, light, and peace. Feasting on the sensual nature of this world now makes me feel as if I'm choosing between two delicious meals and I can't decide which is better. That being said, I won't give up this world easily.

Operation Zero Deductible Going down in Flames
Thursday, January 17, 2013, 8:29 p.m.

Operation Zero Deductible is going down in flames. SOS! Repeat—abort Operation Zero Deductible!

Anyone who has ever worked with me knows I'm a planner, a double-checker, an i dotter, and a t crosser—to an annoying degree. I need to really understand the rules before I start on a project. So when I undertook Operation Zero Deductible, I worked hard to make sure everything was perfect. I spent hours on the phone with the insurance company, the drug company, and the clinic to confirm and reconfirm. I thought it was a sure thing. Then today I found out that even though the drug injection (which the drug company agreed to pay for) was the very first medical treatment I received this year, that clinic didn't submit the bill to the insurance company until after a different clinic for my second treatment of the year submitted. If you're not following, it's because it's so complicated. The bottom line is this: I'll still have to pay part of my deductible. At best, I'll only have to pay six hundred; at worst, I'll have to pay the whole three thousand. Lesson learned—if it seems too good to be true, it probably is.

This all sucks on a financial level, but on an emotional level, it's even worse. When I saw the opportunity to save three thousand dollars on our deductible, I took on the project because it was something I could do to save money for my family. Now it looks like I've failed, which makes me question what I can really contribute to my family.

In others news . . . my boobs glow. I'm not kidding, they *glow*. We realized it today when the sun shone through the window and caught me in just the right way and Wade saw it. You know when you put a flashlight up to your hand and it looks all red? And you can see the veins? It's like that with my (fake) boobs. In the throes of my frustration and deductible disappointment, this miracle ray of sun came through the window. I went into the bathroom, turned off the lights, and tested the phenomenon by shining a flashlight on each breast—*glowing*! Wade seems to think it's cool. My plastic surgeon never told me about this little bonus.

The other good news is that my white count and platelet levels are still low—but now they're on the low side of normal, which is a big improvement. Plus, my tumor markers are down. I started more radiation this week, and it will end next week. Perhaps my whole body will soon be glowing!

Mission Status Change: Operation Two-Thirds Deductible
Friday, January 25, 2013, 2:09 p.m.

Some encouraging things have happened. First, a very nice man from my health insurance company was able to reprocess the bills. He spent four? six? eight? hours making phone calls and working internally on my behalf to help make sure two-thirds of my deductible will be covered by the drug company. While it's not the full amount, it's still a big savings. I need to find a polite way to call my clinic billing office to say, "Don't screw this up again. I have my eyes on you." Then again, maybe I don't need to be so polite all the time.

I'm sure we could all write a book on the nightmares of dealing with our health insurance. It was so encouraging to find someone helpful from the insurance company; he became a real hero in my eyes.

I'm still burning the candle at both ends, being very active and busy. The day before yesterday was my final radiation treatment. Yesterday I needed a nap, and today I can feel I'm dragging. My body is busy rebuilding the damage from the radiation, and I need to scale back my activities.

Medication Vacation

Thursday, February 7, 2013, 5:55 a.m.

My medication vacation will continue into next month. This was a nice surprise made possible by my blood counts, which are once again normal.

I'm eating anything I want, and I've gained ten pounds since the holidays, but I'm happy for it—I know the weight will come back off once my mouth gets blasted with the Afinitor again.

My tumor markers are down again, which is probably from the radiation. Mid-March, I'll have another scan to make sure the radiated area is in check and to look for any new tumors. That will give my doctor the information he needs to move forward with my treatment.

I've been having some numbness and tingling in my hands and feet. I was worried it signaled really bad news; Karen in my support group had the same sensation in her face when the cancer had moved to her brain. The days before my doctor's visit were hellish. I was convinced that my body was riddled with cancer. It was nearly impossible to sleep. Even with sleeping pills, I still didn't get good rest. At one point, I was weeping and feeling like I'd need to go to the psych ward. It's so difficult to live not knowing what's happening inside my body—to get a positive test result but still know that no test is really reliable.

True story: About ten years ago, I went to a doctor presenting with some issues related to a cough. My dad died of throat cancer (from smoking), so I asked about cancer. The doctor told me, "If you had cancer, you'd know it." When she said that, the cancer was already growing in my breast, and I *didn't* know it. Doctors don't have all the answers, and that can be frightening.

We did get some excellent financial news. The headline—we don't need to sell our house! Turns out, I can withdraw retirement money without the 10 percent penalty normally required for early withdrawals. There isn't a ton of money there, but it would allow us to do some things that I'd like to do while I'm still feeling well. We'll spend the next few months consulting with our financial advisor so we can make thoughtful decisions about enjoying life in the short term while maintaining a life that's sustainable in the long term. Penny pinching will continue on a monthly basis, but some retirement money might allow us to enjoy some fruits of my labor. Either way, it means we can stay in our house instead of selling it!

Sh@#!

Friday, March 8, 2013, 8:30 p.m.

My nurse called with scan results today. My soft tissue is still clear, and the spot they radiated in January is better. However, new spots have shown up in my left femur, right hip, and on L2 and T2 in my spine. I didn't talk to the doctor today, and my appointment is a week away. The nurse put me on a cancellation list, so I might be able to see him sooner. Maybe it's a good thing he didn't move up my appointment. If it was really bad, he would have made time, right?

This news sucks. At this point, I'm not thinking about mortality; I'm thinking about pain and plans. Over the past week, Tylenol and Advil haven't been adequately controlling my pain, so last night, I started Percocet again, and it helped relieve the pain enough for me to sleep. My sleep has been awful for about two weeks, and I keep taking more sleep medications. Last night, I realized it was pain waking me up and keeping me awake. The Percocet helps but doesn't take away the pain totally, and it makes me sleepy once daytime rolls around. It's fine for night and naps, but it limits my ability to drive, which means I can't use Percocet just any old time. Having pain again is such a drag. Anyone who has had chronic pain knows how much it controls your life.

Adjustment

Thursday, March 14, 2013, 6:37 p.m.

My adjustment to "one day at a time" is going well. The most difficult part is letting go of thinking about places I'd like to visit with the kids. We've been talking about several trips, including this spring to Sanibel

Island, but I just need to wait and see if I will have the energy to consider future travel.

When a thought about the future pops into my mind, I acknowledge it and say, "I can't pay attention to you right now, because I'm in this moment. I'll attend to you later." It's not unlike how to deal with unruly children.

Speaking of children, I was just interrupted by Jackson. He needed me to play the new Legos board game he invented today. His invented games are pretty cool, and he's such a good little instructor. As he'd promised, the game only took five minutes, and now I'm back.

Yesterday, I met with my lymphedema doctor and therapist. It's been difficult to stay on top of it, but they're pleased with my progress. The swelling has moved into my shoulder, and that's just how it's going to be, but it does respond well to the MLD (manual lymph drainage) and the bandages.

My focus is mostly on the basics: eating, drinking water, pain management, and sleep. Then maybe I'll do one additional thing each day— like today I went to my cancer support group, which is a wonderful source of comfort and care. Other days, I'll return one phone call or write my bills. Just one thing is all I can expect of myself each day. If I do more, it's a bonus.

Sanibel Island, Here We Come

Friday, March 15, 2013, 12:10 p.m.

The visit with Dr. Anderson was a bit rushed because the oncology office seems to be understaffed. He did have enough time to explain that radiation isn't a good option now because the bone mets (bone metastases—I love that my cancer has a nickname) are in so many spots and because we've already radiated several areas. I think too much radiation becomes a problem because the bone marrow can't keep up with its work when too many areas are compromised by radiation.

With radiation out of the picture, we have two options. The first option is to try the Afinitor again, this time with an aromatase inhibitor, and hope it works. While this treatment isn't very different from what I was on when the mets started up again, it could work because the cancer itself has probably mutated. The cancer will continue to mutate, growing resistant to treatment as time goes on.

The second option is Faslodex. Like the others, it blocks the estrogen. The estrogen is what feeds my cancer, so we're essentially trying to starve it. Dr. Anderson thinks this is the best way to go. And if it doesn't work, we can do the Afinitor again. Either way, I'll be keeping my hair—yay! So today I got bone juice in the arm and two Faslodex shots in the butt— both sides. My butt still smarts, despite changing into loose boxer shorts after Wade and I indulged in a big breakfast after the appointment.

Dr. Anderson wants an MRI of my thoracic spine (between the shoulder blades). I've been having pain there, the mets are back in that area, and I've been having some numbness and tingling in my hands and feet. He needs to make sure that nothing is pressing on my spinal cord. I didn't know that was a possibility, and it stinks to have one more thing to worry about.

He also needs an X ray of my hips to make sure the structure of the bones isn't compromised. If the bone looks bad enough, they'll install a metal rod to keep it together. Sounds like a terrible operation, but how cool is it that it's even possible? Living with cancer has made me realize that medicine is a creative endeavor. God is an amazing creator—just look at nature—and then to think he instilled us with brains capable of such creativity. These medical advances feel like God working through people to make the world a better place.

We were cleared for our trip to Sanibel Island in Florida next week, which is a huge relief. This will be the third time we've tried to go in the past few years. Knock on wood that we'll be able to make it. We used our credit-card points to pay for all but one ticket. Dr. Anderson did say that we shouldn't plan any additional vacations yet. He wants to see the MRI and look at my next PET/CT scan, which will happen in another month or two. Once we know how the treatment is working, then we'll be able to decide if travel is safe and smart.

I'm back to "one day at a time" and "be where your hands are" in order to find joy and comfort in all of this uncertainty. I'm so grateful my college humanities teacher included *Man's Search for Meaning* by Viktor Frankl on a syllabus. In it, Frankl, a psychiatrist who lived through the Holocaust, explains we can't choose what happens in life, but we can choose how we react. From that book, I learned we decide how to react when the s#%t hits the fan.

Born to Be Tan

Tuesday, April 9, 2013, 7:45 p.m.

Before leaving on vacation, we learned the MRI looks good. Nothing is pressing on my spinal cord, and my hips and femur aren't in any immediate danger of fracture. Whew.

I can't say enough good things about Sanibel Island. The white beach has beautiful shells. The bay was perfect for fishing and paddleboarding. We spent an afternoon fishing on a boat.

Our one-bedroom cottage was just 350 square feet. Jackson and Vivian were great sports about sleeping on the living room pullout sofa.

I kept thinking we could live somewhere this small—but we were without all the things required for year-round existence. If we didn't need files, insurance records, winter gear, sports gear, musical instruments, pets, Christmas and Halloween decorations, or privacy—perhaps we could make such a small house work. After returning home, our house seems so huge.

We met some wonderful people on Sanibel Island. Let me tell you about just one of them, a Pentecostal vegan health nut with tons of nutritional advice. I'm normally peeved by anyone telling me how to eat, but somehow, she didn't bug me. While most of her advice lacked scientific credentials, she did get through to me on one key point. "You have a serious disease," she said, "and you need to take your nutrition seriously." She also laid her hands on me and prayed. She even started speaking in tongues, which I've not experienced before. While it doesn't follow with my own restrained Episcopal background, her prayers were earnest, and I appreciated the energy and love that she shared.

After we got home, I had my Faslodex shots. A different nurse gave the shots this time, and she put both shots more into my upper butt than into my hips. It hurt for about five days, and it hurt whenever I'd sit or lay on my back. Lesson learned: I'll need to tell the next nurse where to put the shots so I can avoid that prolonged discomfort.

The warm Sanibel Island sun has great healing power. I was born to be tan. Now that I have a little bit of a tan, I look and feel a million times better.

Unhappy Chemo Campers
Thursday, April 11, 2013, 9:29 p.m.

Today was a difficult day. After support group, one of the women pulled me aside to share what I'd missed while in Florida. Karen—whose cancer spread to her brain a few months ago—has been given only one or two months to live.

It's terrible to learn that someone in my own camp has received this terrible news. Karen is positive, kind, and always knows the right thing to say. It's so unfair. She should be here on earth longer. We all joined the group knowing that our membership would change (and shrink) over time, but she's the first among us to be told she only has a few months to live. It doesn't make me more worried about myself, but it does help me understand what you, my friends, may feel when you hear bad news about me.

Non-Cancer Annoyances
Monday, April 22, 2013, 9:49 a.m.

Every now and then, I have the energy to go to Target, but I'm starting to question if it's a good idea. I went yesterday, but then my hip was sore all evening. Clearly, I overdid it. I've been thinking about using a grocery delivery service. Then I can spend my physical energy doing things that don't make me sore.

This morning, something reminded me that cancer doesn't mean I'm immune to other life annoyances. Waking an hour late, at 7:30 a.m., I realized I'd set my alarm for 6:30 *p.m.* instead of *a.m.* My very punctual Vivian was furious that I'd overslept and glared at me as she went to take a shower. Then I went to wake Jackson, who wasn't in his bed, which gave me that momentary panic of "Someone stole my baby!" The little stinker was sitting at the dining room table doing his homework. His very cute first-grade homework. I got him dressed in time to drive Vivian's carpool and get Jackson to his school because he'd missed the bus. Whew.

When I returned home after that harrowing morning, I discovered cat puke on the dining room table and dog pee on the bed. Hope the rest of the day is calmer.

You Never Walk Alone

Wednesday, April 24, 2013, 7:15 p.m.

Can I start by saying something about you, dear reader? Do you understand that if you were in my position, people would surround you with love? Do you understand that people are ready to spring out of nowhere to help you? Hold that message close, because it's true.

If you're walking alone through difficulty, you can ask for help. Not just illness, but worry, grief, or any kind of suffering, I pray there are people who will help you. Based on my experience, you never walk alone.

This week, I want to a healing center called Pathways to attend a class called Forgiveness as a Path to Wholeness. It's a six-week class based on a text called *A Course in Miracles*. The class was very different from what I'd expected. I thought it would focus on recognizing who or what we need to forgive and then getting advice on how to accomplish that. Instead, I learned that fear and love are the only two reactions we have. I learned ways to approach situations in a spirit of love and that we're all innocent and pure at heart. Already, I've broken some negative cycles. It's a lifelong practice, but I'm optimistic that I can become adept at beaming positive energy out to the world.

Tonight, I'm home alone, and I'm going to indulge in time watching TV. Not the best example of beaming positive energy, but I just can't resist—season two of *Breaking Bad* is waiting for me. I'm going to go enjoy some high-quality (and very dark) storytelling and acting. And no matter how bad cancer gets for me, at least I don't have to worry about angry drug dealers coming after me like poor Walter White.

A Day to Remember
Saturday, April 27, 2013, 4:01 p.m.

Yesterday was a day to remember on several fronts. It would have been Mom's eighty-third birthday, so I lit a candle for her, talked to her for a little while, and then had a good cry. Today is the fourth anniversary of her passing.

Right now, Jackson is at a friend's birthday party, and Vivian is at play rehearsal. When they get home, we'll remember my mom with dinner at one of her favorite places, Baker's Square. We'll order our dessert first, as she always did. Starting at a young age, she was able to get her mom to serve dessert first by promising to eat all her dinner, which she would do. As an adult, she'd always order her dessert first at restaurants. It's a fun way for us to remember her today.

We'll also look at some photos of my mom so I can remind my kids of her kindness, sweetness, and humor. I want them to remember that she was a nurse and that she worked in public health for over forty years. She was a tough cookie, but you'd never know it because she was so unassuming. We miss that little lady very much.

A theologian (I'm not sure who) said parents are a child's first glimpse into the face of God. When Mom died, something about my relationship to God dramatically shifted. I didn't feel as connected as I had before. My notion of God is connected to my mom. Now I'm working to improve my relationship with God as the relationship with my mom continues to change.

Yesterday was the first day we hit seventy degrees in this yucky, snowy spring. Today is another sunny and beautiful day to remember my sweet mom.

This Season's Big Color: Orange

Tuesday, April 30, 2013, 7:31 p.m.

As of ten minutes ago, it's officially the warm-weather season. I realized this when a neighbor boy opened the front door and just walked right in, asking, "Where's Jackson?" No knock, no "Hello," no coat to remove, no boots to shake off, just "Where's Jackson?" I love being that house. Kids just walk in without even thinking about knocking. It makes me feel like I'm in a sitcom where the silly neighbor just walks in. Growing up was often lonely with just me and Mom, and now I love having a bustling home.

The color orange seems to define this time in my life. This spring, I've bought two new T-shirts—orange; a new cardigan—orange; painted my finger and toenails—orange. I'm craving oranges, tangerines, peaches, and sweet potatoes—all orange. When choosing a ball for Jackson from the bin of giant bouncy balls, of all the many colors, I picked orange. Lupita's new outfit—orange. New lipstick—orange.

I've been learning an unbelievable amount in the last ten days from so many sources—the forgiveness group at Pathways, church education classes, my church healing circle (which included a Reiki session). My life is changing, and I'm absorbing so much so fast. Through it all, the color orange keeps popping up. When something keeps showing up over and over again, it's time to pay attention.

I've never been very tuned into the chakras other than knowing they existed. But when I had my first Reiki session last week, the practitioner mentioned some blockages at my Sacral Chakra—guess where it is? At my hip / pelvis / L2 vertebrae. The spots where my cancer is most active and where the metastasis and pain began. Coincidence? Even if you're not into this stuff, please stick with me here. All the orange in my life lately? My craving for orange? Turns out one of the ways to heal that chakra is a good dose of orange—eating orange food, wearing orange, looking at orange.

To me, this means that without even knowing it, I'm getting back in tune with my intuition. I've been able to be quiet, listen, and obey my attraction to orange.

Will orange cure my cancer? Statistically unlikely. But does that matter? Not really, because my spirit is lifting. Could it mean more years of life? It doesn't matter, because I'm getting more life out of my years. More life out of each day. Healing is happening on a spiritual level, an emotional level—and if it happens on the physical level, great. But if the physical body doesn't follow, it doesn't matter, because my spirit is feeling lighter.

I've been experiencing deep sorrow about the deadly building collapse in Bangladesh and all the fires that have happened in garment factories there and elsewhere worldwide in the past months. Most workers are girls, an average age of thirteen. With a daughter at that age, I feel deep grief that these girls' lives, like the garments they make, are considered disposable. It's not only inexpensive brands that are involved but Gap and Tommy Hilfiger, among others. I'm going to seek out "Made in the USA" labels from now on. Or just buy less. I'm going to keep saying prayers for those who have died and keep talking about this to other moms. Together, we can deliver a message to this industry that uses young girls as slaves to sew clothing that's then marketed to First World young girls. It's such a sick cycle.

As I become more in tune with myself, the existence of injustice becomes increasingly difficult to tolerate. I remind myself that anger is an unsustainable emotion. It takes way too much energy to continue anger for long periods of time. So now I'm learning to apply love. That conjures up images of applying a medication to skin, applying a bandage to a wound, applying a warm compress to a sore spot. Love is about healing.

So I'm not changing my buying habits out of anger for the working conditions; I'm doing it for love of the workers. The argument that we can only save our economy by buying the goods that are being produced in a cruel manner doesn't hold up. Businesses operate on a quarterly cycle, and if consumers stop buying what they're selling, it will speed up the process for business to adjust to what consumers demand.

Please bear with me as I keep learning. When we try new things, we're often clumsy, and I trust you to tolerate and apply love to my new wisdom. May others apply love to you, as well.

Ten Little Monkeys

Monday, May 6, 2013, 7:12 p.m.

We had Jackson's seventh birthday starring ten little monkey men running wild in the backyard. They had such fun, and nobody was injured, which seems like a miracle. Jackson announced at dinner tonight that three girls like him. He's turning out to be an amazing little guy and a ladies' man to boot.

Last night, I dreamed my lymphedema went away. Just woke up one morning and my right arm was the same size as my left. Poof, just like that. It was a wonderful dream. In real life, I have exercises to do, a Flexitouch machine that assists with lymphatic drainage, and unsightly compression garments that I must wear twenty-two hours a day. It's been really bothering me to spend so much time on my arm when it isn't getting better. It's only maintaining at one to three centimeters larger than my left. I worry that it's going to become even more difficult to find clothing that fits both my normal left arm and my enlarged right arm. If only the lymphedema and the cancer would just disappear like in my dream. But in our waking lives, I guess we just problem-solve and find ways to make our circumstances work. I'm already looking forward to going to sleep tonight. Wishing to dream about wholeness again.

Another Scan Planned
Friday, May 10, 2013, 7:44 p.m.

Today, Wade and I went to my oncology appointment expecting: an Xgeva (bone) shot in the arm, two Faslodex (hormone) shots in the butt, a visit with the doctor, and needing to schedule a scan for June. Because I reported pain in my hips, back, and ribs, the scan got bumped up to next week, and they postponed the Faslodex. We decided to see if it's working before I get another treatment.

I'm trying to enjoy not having pain in my butt from the Faslodex shots, but I'm nervous about the scan results. My doctor's gut feeling is that I'm responding well and that we'll just need to find some new ways to manage my pain more effectively.

He gave me a new prescription for pain, but my goal is to move away from narcotics because they aren't providing the consistent relief I need. They're fine for bedtime, but I have reservations about taking them during the day. No need to add a driving-while-intoxicated charge to my list of problems.

To keep my mind off the scan, I'm looking forward to a new bottle of silver nail polish. In Florida, I saw several sets of silver toenails, and it looked so cute I resolved to carry the trend north.

Best Mother's Day Ever
Sunday, May 12, 2013, 10:27 p.m.

This morning we went to church, and then I slept for three hours in the afternoon. We followed our tradition of buying flowers for our front-step pots on Mother's Day. We also bought lettuce, spinach, chard, and beet plants. Wade and Vivian rebuilt the backyard window boxes for our greens. The bunnies can't get to the lettuce in a window box. Wade rebuilt our garden beds, and they look great. In a single day, Wade installed an irrigation system, so now our trees and veggie beds can be watered by simply turning on the spout.

Vivian uncomplainingly helped Wade in the garden, and Jackson insisted on making lunch for me. I helped him a little, but only by turning on the stove and cutting the veggies. He washed the tomatoes and carrots, poured the pasta into the water, put the oil in the pan, and buttered the bread for garlic toast. He is a wonderful little cook and so sweet to insist on doing everything himself.

Jackson gave me two wonderful gifts—one was a card he made in Spanish class that was all about me. He was so sweet reading in Spanish and translating for me. The other was a picture he drew of me along with the following list in English:

> My mom is: funny
> My mom is: cool
> My mom's hair is: soft
> My mom is: nice
> My mom is: interested in anything

Mother's Day doesn't get much better than that.

Today's Scan

Monday, May 13, 2013, 9:00 p.m.

Today's PET/CT scan was uneventful. I've got drinking the nasty chalky stuff down to a science. Use two straws, hold my nose, and gulp as quickly as possible. No more fussing about drinking it. Just get it over with.

In the waiting room, I spied a magazine I've not seen before: *Practical Pain Management*. The cover article was on cancer pain. Normally, I avoid cancer magazines. It's bad enough I'm spending my time hanging out in nasty waiting rooms; I'd much rather read about something fun, like fashion, hairstyles, or makeup.

Practical Pain Management was better than a fashion magazine. What I've learned in just a few articles hits home with me. It confirmed what Dr. Anderson said last week: "We need to know the source of the pain to know how to treat it." I've also started to take the psychological impact of pain more seriously. The magazine article stated that emotional pain can affect the same regions of the brain as physical pain, and it cites research that shows depression and post-traumatic stress disorder are both common in people with cancer. The article also describes several types of pain, including mine, perfectly: constant, aching, gnawing.

Wade and I think my pain threshold has probably gone up since the original diagnosis. Dealing with pain on a daily basis means I notice it less, but that doesn't make the effects of the pain less problematic. In fact, it might make them worse, because I'm better at ignoring pain, when perhaps I'd be doing better if I made a commitment to treating it.

The bottom line of the magazine's articles is that poor pain management can be deadly. From my own firsthand experience with pain, I can see how that's true. When I was in so much pain after surgeries and during chemo, I felt it would be OK if my life ended. Those thoughts seemed rational at the time because I just wanted the pain to stop. But after cancer treatment, it would seem a terrible pity for someone to die of suicide.

The first step is to embrace the knowledge that pain is real, and it can be treated—and this magazine gave me hope it can be treated.

Fair to Partly Cloudy

Wednesday, May 15, 2013, 7:13 p.m.

My nurse called today with scan results. The areas with the bone metastases look worse than the last scan. It's not the news I wanted, but it's better than hearing that new areas are lighting up. Dr. Anderson will change my medication, because the Faslodex isn't doing the job.

I'm glad I reported the pain. Had I ignored it, he would have waited another month for my scan. I'm proud of myself for asking my pain, "What are you trying to tell me?" Asking that simple question means we'll start a new treatment a full month earlier than we would have if I'd run away from the pain.

Since reading *Practical Pain Management*, I've been able to calm down and feel less afraid. Now that I know the physical pain and the emotional distress are in the same part of the brain, I can avoid panic when I feel the pain, which in turn makes the pain less pronounced.

Cancer is a big bunch of poop. Not a cute little Tootsie Roll–sized Lupita Maria Chihuahua poop, but a giant Labrador retriever poop.

I'm going to chill out and watch the most recent episode of *Call the Midwife* while snuggling my little Lupita Maria. It will help me get a good night's sleep so I can face tomorrow with intelligence and love.

Tantrum

Thursday, May 16, 2013, 8:34 p.m.

At the oncology clinic today, Wade and I were presented with two drug options: Xeloda (an oral chemo I've not tried yet) or Afinitor combined with Aromasin. We decided to go with Xeloda. The main side effects will be red, peeling hands, fatigue, mouth sores, and diarrhea. Sounds like a party!

It was so difficult to decide between the two drug options. We don't know how well either will work. It was a stressful decision because neither will cure me; they'll just buy me more time. Don't get me wrong; I'm happy to buy more time, but it kind of makes me feel like I lose no matter what I decide. The nurse assured me that we have more drugs to try if these don't work, but today it was hitting home that as we cross ineffective drugs off the list, there are fewer left to try. Often I feel cancer is just a small part of my life, but today it felt much bigger, and I hate it.

Another thing that depressed me was asking about getting more radiation. Turns out there's a lifetime limit because you need a certain amount of undamaged bone marrow to survive, and the radiation damages the marrow. Not sure if I'm close to that limit, but it was another reminder that there are fewer options as time goes on, which makes me mad.

After we left oncology office, we walked over to the hospital for an X ray to make sure my femur is still strong. On the walk over, I felt like a toddler having a temper tantrum. I just wanted to hit and kick something and cry and say, "No!" to everything. Wade talked me down off the ledge. I'm mad. I wish the cancer could be personified outside my body so I could just poop on it and kill it with my poop. Poop, poop, poop. Yes, I'm acting like a baby. I hate cancer. It's stupid and ugly, and I want to beat it up. I want it gone, gone, gone. Stupid. Poop.

Wade said we could get a punching bag so I could really have a temper tantrum. But that would just make my lymphedema worse. Poop.

Surprise Party
Saturday, May 18, 2013, 10:57 p.m.

Wow—today we attended three parties! The first was a Chihuahua Party that I created and hosted as part of Vivian's school fund-raiser. Five parent-child pairs enjoyed Chihuahua-themed cupcakes, playing with Lupita, and photos with Lupita. We watched funny Chihuahua videos on YouTube. The best part was Lupita strutting her stuff on the catwalk (a.k.a. our dining room table) modeling her favorite outfits to fashion show music. It was cute and fun.

We also went to Vivian's cast party, which was held at the playwright's house. It was fun but also sad because it signals the end of the show's run tomorrow. Vivian is always sad when a show ends, but she takes it all in stride. She knows she'll forever have her castmates as friends. Plus, there's always another play around the corner.

The party in between those two parties was the most amazing of all three: a Spring Is Finally Here party across the street. When we got there, I noticed many people wearing orange. I thought, *Wow, it really must be the color of the season!* Then our neighbor announced they were all wearing orange in response to my recent CaringBridge orange entry. The orange was to honor me—I loved it! All the plates, napkins, and table coverings were orange too. What a kind thing to do; I was amazed at their thoughtfulness. Then our neighbors presented us with a lovely floral arrangement with a dozen envelopes within the arrangement. He said I've written about wanting to make family memories and this is a gift to help us do that.

The four of us opened the envelopes to discover awesome gifts, including gift cards, art and history museum memberships, and theater tickets. Then our neighbor gave us one more gift—a novelty-sized check for an incredibly generous amount of money to help us fund ways to make memories together.

It took about twenty minutes of me talking to people and telling them thank you to realize the party was planned for us—the neighborhood party to welcome spring was a ruse. We were so blown away. And thankful. We have a great community! The gifts and money were wonderful, but as I told my neighbors, that they wore orange in support of me was more than enough to lift my spirit.

Gloves and Safety Glasses
Monday, May 20, 2013, 6:43 p.m.

The Xeloda arrived in the mail today. I'm grateful to have health insurance. I'm grateful to be receiving this treatment. Now that the obligatory gratitude over, I'll commence with the complaining.

Always the A+ student, I read all the manufacturer's information sheets with new drugs. I used to just laugh at these crazy side effect information sheets, but after experiencing so many of the side effects, I know they're no laughing matter. This information sheet freaked me out. "It is recommended to use GLOVES and SAFETY GLASSES to avoid exposure in case a tablet breaks. If powder from a broken tablet comes into contact with skin, wash skin immediately with soap and water. If powder comes into contact with your mouth, nose, or eyes, rinse thoroughly with water." And they want me to *swallow* six of these pills daily?! OK, I guess it's kind of funny in an absurdist way, but it scared me when I first read it. Needless to say, I didn't wear gloves or safety glasses to take my first dose.

I'm convinced the drug company lawyers had way too much time on their hands and added gloves and safety glasses into the information sheet for purely legal reasons. It's the same lawyerly phenomenon that causes some peanut butter jars to have this warning: "Made in a facility that processes peanuts."

Pooped
Tuesday, May 28, 2013, 4:02 p.m.

I did absolutely nothing over the weekend. The side effects from Xeloda are really kicking in now that I've been on it for a week. The nausea is manageable, but the fatigue has me completely wiped out, and my fingers are becoming raw and painful. The quality of my sleep changed after the first few days of Xeloda. It's a deeper sleep, even when I nap during the day. But it isn't a restful sleep. When I am awake, I'm less alert than I was with the Faslodex. If I even think about doing something like cleaning the kitchen or writing bills, I get totally overwhelmed and don't know where to begin, as if those things were climbing a mountain that required supplies, maps, a strategy, and so on. It's awful when small tasks seem insurmountable. I've totally lost interest in most TV shows. Keeping a little food in my stomach helps with the nausea, so I'm focusing on eating a little here and there.

Jackson just came into my room to show me a new TV show he likes, so watching TV with him is going to have to count for "doing something" today!

Bad Grass Is Hard to Kill
Sunday, June 2, 2013, 9:46 p.m.

This weekend was so much better than last weekend. I started feeling better midweek. Wade figured out that maybe I had a little bug over the weekend. It never occurs to either of us that I can actually get sick—as in normal sick. Not everything can be blamed on cancer medications. One thing that provided hope last week was taking all my Xeloda out of the bottle to count the pills to see how many were left before my week off from it. I take six per day, and it was fun to count the pills left in the bottle and confirm that my final dose will be tomorrow morning. Then I'll have a full week off from Xeloda before starting the next fourteen days of pills.

My fingers aren't hurting anymore, just a shadow of the sensation I was feeling when I first started. My nausea is better as long as I keep a little something in my stomach. My fatigue is letting up. Maybe this medication won't be so bad—I know that after a few cycles it may be a different story, but I'll take feeling OK for now.

Tonight at dinner, we saw Ray, a family friend from the Philippines. He also has Stage IV cancer and was told he'd die a few years ago. He's the sole survivor from his clinical trial group. Each time he's in Minnesota, we compare notes on cancer. This time, he provided a great little gem—"Bad grass is hard to kill." He said it sounds much better in Spanish and Filipino, but I love it in English, as well. I'm going to imagine myself as a weed that just keeps on going and going. Nobody can get rid of me!

We also talked about laughter and how it's a secret of our survival. I need to remember laughter when I'm starting to feel depressed. The next time checking my e-mail or loading the dishwasher is too overwhelming, maybe I can laugh a little to chase away feeling overwhelmed. There must be videos of stand-up comedy that I can find on my phone. I've long thought stand-up comedy is the highest art. To stand on stage and try to make people laugh is the definition of bravery.

Wade has been working hard on improving the backyard by building a deck next to the pond and putting a wood floor in the garage. He'll soon bring his pottery supplies out to the garage so he can get his studio out of the basement for the summer months. It will be nice to have him working there in the afternoons, and hopefully the kids can play by the pond without bothering him too much.

Saturday was a triumph for me because I went to a festival in downtown Saint Paul with Vivian. We walked about eight blocks, and I didn't feel sore. The walking was slow and just a block or two at a time—but still, it was a big deal. It gives me hope about participating in some of the fun things I want to do this summer. It also gives me hope that Xeloda is working. And if it's just a placebo effect, I'll take it, because I love to walk.

A Good Tired

Tuesday, June 11, 2013, 11:44 a.m.

Yesterday, Dr. Anderson finally gave me a good report. All my numbers look great. Even my cholesterol and triglycerides are getting back to normal. So much so that he's eliminating the cholesterol medication for a few weeks to see how I manage without it.

My tumor markers will be available tomorrow. I'll be surprised if they're moving in the wrong direction. He was happy to hear that my level of pain is decreased. It's a sign that Xeloda is working.

During my weeklong medication vacation (which is now over, sadly) my cousin Kristin, my closest childhood relative, was in town. She lives in New York State, but we grew up seeing each other pretty much every summer. We were able to spend more time together than most other visits. She mentioned remembering the time early in her life when she "became Kristin." I've been reflecting on the time in late elementary school and early middle school when I started to understand who I was, what I cared about, what I embraced, and what I rejected. Spending time with Kristin helped me reconnect with that person I was becoming at that early age. So often, I look back with regret that my life turned out so differently from what I had planned. (Who on earth has things turn out as they'd planned?)

Kristin and I stayed up late and attended Northern Spark. It's a dusk-to-dawn art event. We followed a procession with an East Indian dance troupe. We stumbled upon individual artists presenting their multimedia projects. We experienced our first art-cart gallery, which was a dollhouse-sized, Plexiglas-encased miniature art gallery. I want one! We participated in interactive performance art. While all the walking made me really sore, and I had to take breaks to sit, it was worth it, because I ran into many people I haven't seen for years.

The highlight of the evening was a writer's brawl. Two writers were given a prompt and had fifteen minutes to think about it. Then they had fifteen minutes to write—on circa 1980s typewriters—in front of a crowd, with musicians and dancers trying to distract them the entire time. The pieces they read out loud were wonderful. Although Northern Spark went until dawn, we were home by 11:30 p.m. Still, I left feeling I'd experienced something really unique. Our early departure gave us plenty of time to stay up late and talk, just like we did as kids.

The night was a gift from our friend Irene, who bravely took both of my kids for a sleepover. It was wonderful to have a full night off from being a parent. I also had the night off from being a wife because Wade is up north fishing with friends. We can't really call or text reliably, so he's been calling each evening from a spot where he has cell phone reception. When I asked how the accommodations were, he gushed, "We had to boat in. We're twelve miles from any road. We're the only ones here except the owners—it's just great."

To me, that sounds like hell on earth because it seems a perfect place for serial killers to hang out, but hey, I'm glad he's having fun! Before he left, he pulled up the website, which showed nothing but trees, water, and men holding large fish. Wade pointed at the screen, saying, "Doesn't it look wonderful?"

Not to me. I'd feel too far out of my element to relax, what with the lurking serial killers and all. Not only that, I need the city lights to be calm.

Father's Day
Sunday, June 16, 2013, 11:06 a.m.

Today is a good day. Wade is home from fishing. It's still impossible for me to understand how standing on a boat all day with a fishing pole is relaxing, but he's clearly relaxed and happy. Jackson is so excited that it's Father's Day. He's been planning to make pancakes and help Dad all day long. He even made a card and created a gift out of his own treasures—coral from Florida, polished rocks, part of his own treasured kneaded eraser, and a dime. Seven-year-olds are the best! Of course, Wade loved his gifts. Vivian made a card with a cute poem. She wanted to buy him a Japanese red maple tree, but I insisted we wait until we could discuss it with Wade because it will involve moving other plants. So instead, we'll visit the garden store and probably get more plants for the pond instead.

The kids and I also gave him the one thing he really wanted—an antelope skull, presented with the caveat that it go in the garage or basement. It's a lovely object, but I don't want to look at it while I'm eating dinner. Wade's collection of small skulls (bird, rodent, monkey) doesn't bug me, but a giant skull isn't what I want to look at all the time. I'd prefer to see Wade's paintings in our living room.

I love to spend a day celebrating what a good dad Wade is to our kids. He teaches them about nature, drawing, carpentry, art, fixing things, and being a good neighbor. But the lead-up to Father's Day was crap for me. In the last few days, the Xeloda side effects have been mostly nausea. Before Wade came home from his fishing trip, I had to drive Vivian to an outdoor opera and a musical—in both cases, I had to drop her with her friends so I could go home and rest. Barfing in the car was a distinct possibility both times but luckily didn't happen.

The Other Side of the Waiting Room
Wednesday, June 19, 2013, 3:04 p.m.

What a crazy few days we've had. Today, I'm sitting on the other side of the waiting room while Wade has surgery on his hand. On Monday, he was doing some woodwork in the garage. I was just outside it deadheading irises. I was thinking about what a beautiful day it was and what a luxury it is to deadhead flowers—thinking life was feeling a little more in control. Then I heard Wade swear—not an uncommon sound when he's working in the garage—but this was different, so I dropped everything to see him shaking his arm.

His left thumb, just above the top knuckle, had been nearly cut off by the table saw. The top was hanging by a flap of skin. We drove directly to the ER. Luckily, both of the kids were still in their day camps.

I wasn't able to even look at his hand, so I kept my back to him in the ER, while he texted bloody pictures to his friends. I caught a quick glimpse, and it's all I needed. The ER staff was amazing. They cleaned him up, gave him fourteen stitches, and sent him home with antibiotics and pain meds. They referred him to a hand surgeon, knowing he'd need more treatment to keep the thumb.

As I waited for my car at the ER valet station, a man hopped in leaning on the arm of his friend (he clearly had a painful foot injury). Then a very pregnant woman came in with her mom and husband. Clearly she was in terrible pain. An extremely distressed mother in slippers carried her baby in from a taxicab. It was heartbreaking to witness so much pain in such a short amount of time. I'm sure ER doctors and nurses are trained to keep their emotions at bay, but I felt like a puddle after seeing Wade's pain, much less the parade of other miserable people. I could easily get swept up in all that suffering. Hopefully, they're all doing much better today.

After we returned home, I hurried to the backyard to clean up the trail of blood before the kids got home. I felt like Walter White in *Breaking Bad* as I hosed off the bloody patio and garage floor. The song playing in my head the whole time was from a *Thomas the Tank Engine* movie, "Accidents happen, now and again, when you least expect . . . just when you think that life is OK, fate comes to collect." The creepy juxtaposition of a toddler song while cleaning up a bloody mess really made it seem like a *Breaking Bad* moment. Granted, cleaning up thumb-injury blood isn't the same as the "accidents" Walt cleans up on *Breaking Bad*, but it still made me feel like I had more than inoperable cancer in common with poor Walt.

We met with the hand surgeon yesterday, who said this isn't an unusual injury or a complicated case. They think Wade's thumb can be saved, but it will depend on how he heals. The bone was shattered. We could see the fragments on the X ray. Gnarly.

So today I sit in the waiting room—and it's weird. Wade even almost said my birth date when they asked for his, because we're both so conditioned to having me as the patient. The surgery is using a local nerve block, and Wade was happy to have his thumb numbed up as they prepared for surgery. Despite narcotics, ice packs, and elevation, he's still been experiencing a lot of pain. Even moving his arm hurts because the nerves are connected all the way up his arm down into the thumb. I hope the surgery will resolve both his pain and improve his range of motion.

When he gets home today, he'll have a few merciful hours until the block wears off, so hopefully he can enjoy being pain-free for a little while.

Luckily, it was his left hand, so he should be able to throw pottery again. However, it will be six to eight weeks before he's able to resume work and normal activity. Wade thinks he'll be back to work within a week, but based on his pain level and what the doctor has said, I doubt even Wade's midwestern work ethic will outpace the doctor's estimate. He'll have to keep his hands dry for two weeks until the skin heals and then another two weeks for the incisions to heal once the screws are removed. Pottery-making involves wet hands all day long, with lots o' germs lurking in the water. This means until the incision heals completely, he'll have to keep out of clay. Wade thinks he'll be able to do some other type of work at the pottery shop, but he's going to discover for himself that pain management is a full-time job.

Wade is worried about cash flow because he doesn't have disability insurance, but this is exactly why we have emergency savings. I have no problem dipping into it if we need to replace some of his income over the next few weeks.

The surgeon just came in and said Wade did well. He had to shorten the thumb a little, and Wade will have three pins in his hand for six weeks. I'm glad Wade is doing well, but six weeks is a long time.

Overdue Update

Tuesday, July 2, 2013, 12:30 p.m.

The last two weeks have been eventful. Wade's thumb is healing well. He spent a week on narcotic painkillers until our wise pharmacist neighbor suggested the maximum dose of Advil, which actually worked even better than the narcotics. The switch also allowed him to drive again.

My Xeloda side effects have remained pretty consistent—pain in my hands and now the soles of my feet, tummy trouble, and fatigue. The fatigue is the worst. Even though I've been experiencing fatigue for so long, I still find it difficult to describe. It's not like being tired after running a long distance or the feeling you have just before nodding off to sleep.

Fatigue is a heaviness that weighs the mind and body, enveloping all consciousness. Fatigue can't be relieved by a cup of coffee, cold water, or a positive attitude. Fatigue is not negotiable. It's like a diabetic reaction—but I have yet to find fatigue's insulin. One would think sleep would revive a fatigued person, but sleep doesn't always come easily. Only rest, sometimes sleep, and the passage of time seem to temporarily relieve fatigue.

One recent discovery is something that has been suggested to me for years—ginger. Aside from being my favorite *Gilligan's Island* castaway, I've enjoyed ginger in sweet treats like gingersnaps, ginger ale, and so on. But I think raw ginger root tastes awful. So whenever anyone would suggest chewing on ginger to relieve fatigue, I balked. Then my neighbor gave me a bottle of crystallized ginger from her cupboard because I'd mentioned nausea. I'm amazed to report two things: First, it doesn't taste gross—it's covered in sugar and is like chewing a little piece of candy. Second, it has completely relieved my nausea. I'm amazed and so happy to know how to control at least one incredibly disruptive symptom.

The experience with ginger inspired me to seek other alternative treatments. For example, I had my first acupuncture session yesterday. My top goal is to get pain relief so I can move more. It's too soon to know how well it will work, but the session itself wasn't as bad as I'd anticipated. The acupuncture needles are so small that they only hurt for a moment. There was one needle in my hand that I asked her to remove because it continued to feel spicy even after a few minutes. Other than that, it was pretty easy. I have two more sessions in the upcoming two weeks. If I see some positive results, I'll find out if my health insurance will cover additional sessions.

My tolerance for pain and discomfort is very low these days. Even hearing swearing or negative news stories hurts my soul. My emotional rawness is partly due to some disturbing events in the life of my support group. The upside to a support group is a room full of people who totally "get it" from a firsthand perspective. They give incredibly meaningful advice. It's an opportunity to help others in my same boat. The downside is that this disease only gets worse. Yes, there are temporary successes, but we all know we're on an unhappy trajectory.

I've written a while back about Karen from my support group; the cancer spread to her brain a few months ago. The treatment is really hard on her, but if she stops treatment, she'll become blind and unable to move. It's unknown if the treatment will extend her life. Her prognosis is several months. Another support group member has also been told her cancer moved to her brain. She's in the early stages of treatment and didn't ask her doctor for a prognosis because she should have died four years ago, so she's happy with any extra time she has.

The sadness of seeing these two beautiful women, both moms, meet our ultimate fear is indescribable. It seems impossible that no one has figured out how to beat this disease. I feel sad, angry, and most of all, afraid. We talk as a group about how we want to support those whose disease has progressed, but it's terrifying to see your own disease play out in a cherished friend's body. Karen lost her ability to drive due to seizures caused by her brain metastasis. Being unable to drive is such a major loss of freedom.

Perhaps the most disturbing part of these cases of brain metastasis is this: both women had seemingly minor symptoms. One had a slight numbness in her jaw, the other became able to "see her pulse" when she was looking at a blank field, such as a white wall. Both of these are things that might go unsaid at a doctor's visit, and I'm so grateful that both spoke up and were able to get early intervention, giving them time to say their good-byes.

Once again, I'm remembering the phrase: "Be where your hands are." I understand that to mean staying in the present moment is the best remedy for me right now.

Staying in the moment is great in theory, but we also need to plan. I have some travel I'd like to do with my family, and it's time to start making plans, but that's scary when I'm not sure what new treatment is around the corner. The travel plans won't happen today, so I'm going to set my fears aside and do the things that need to get done—laundry, phone calls for the kids' activities, and painting my fingernails red, white, and blue for the upcoming holiday.

Best Fourth Ever

Sunday, July 7, 2013, 3:07 p.m.

Our Fourth of July was wonderful. It was a perfect Minnesota day. We spent the afternoon in our backyard. The fireworks in our neighborhood park were the best ever—I sat with Jackson in my lap, and we talked the whole time about each firework.

The next day, I imposed forced child labor. We have millions of weeds along the side garden, and I decided we needed to annihilate them. Wade hoed, Vivian and Jackson complained and cried, and I yelled. In the midst of this ruckus, I saw a creature that looked like a blind chipmunk run past me. Wade said, "Catch it!" So I did. It was a baby bunny that hadn't even opened its eyes yet. It was so darling! Then, right where I caught it, we noticed a nest—with *five* more bunnies! The cutest ever! We all got to pick them up and snuggle and talk to them in high-pitched, squeaky voices. Then we put them back in the nest and finished our weeding.

I told the children it was a good lesson because if I wouldn't have forced them to pull weeds, we never would have found the bunnies. It's a good lesson that even when things seem bleak, cuteness can be found. That night, we went to Melissa and Uri's house for more celebrating and more fireworks.

Vivian loves playing their grand piano, so it didn't surprise me when she called me over to listen to her play. What did surprise me is that she sang while she played! She's been working on learning the piano part for "Someone Like You" by Adele. As she played and sang, I totally started to cry. Then she played for Wade, and we both cried. Just as the fireworks were about to start, she assembled a group of around ten of my cousin Alexa's twentysomething med-school friends to listen to her perform it again. As she played, my cousin Melissa and I held hands and cried. I felt so proud of her piano skills, beautiful voice, and assembling an audience. She's an amazing little lady.

Along with all the fun we've had with the bunnies, songs, late nights, and fireworks during the last few days, I've managed my fatigue by sleeping until two in the afternoon the other day and taking my first nap at 11:00 a.m. today. When I'm having fun during awake times, it makes all the sleeping and resting worthwhile.

Shu Shu is snuggling on the bed with me now, and Lupita Maria is at my side. Jackson just came in with a wicked cool paper airplane, and Vivian is patiently waiting for me to take her to Target. It's nearly 3:00 p.m., so it's time to finally take a shower and use up my energy for another day with my family.

Happy Scan
Thursday, July 18, 2013, 8:10 p.m.

My PET/CT scan came back with the best possible result—the cancer is considerably less active than it was on the last scan. This is great news because it means less cancer, plus I'll stay on the Xeloda. The side effects are annoying, but I can live with them. I'd rather stay with the devil I know than face the devil I don't know.

I'm also happy to report that I've been over a week with no Percocet at night and no sleeping medication. My quality of sleep is better, as well. Walking up the block and walking more in stores must be helping reset my sleep cycle. I still need lorazepam to get to sleep, but it feels great to have cut two drugs from my repertoire. It's possible I'll need them in the future, but for now, I'm enjoying fewer pills, less hip pain, and more freedom to move.

So many other good things are happening lately. Jackson and I had a wonderful little "date" on Friday night at the science museum, Saturday we barbecued with friends, Sunday my healing circle was wonderful, Monday I had acupuncture, and Tuesday Wade and I celebrated nineteen years of marriage. Plus, this whole week we've harvested a big bowl of raspberries each day.

The emotional roller coaster continues, up and down each day. Now that I have another three months before my next scan, I can set the anxiety aside—knock on wood that I don't get a headache or some weird symptom that triggers an earlier scan. My focus now is finding the right complementary treatments to go along with my oncology care. I've scheduled more acupuncture and a monthly massage. After successfully using ginger to help my nausea, I've also started to use lavender to help me sleep. Realizing it's been months since I've seen my counselor, I've scheduled some sessions. She'll help me deal with seeing my support group friends who are progressing in their disease. More Reiki sessions are also in my future. In September, I'll attend a four-day retreat for women with metastatic breast cancer. I'm filling my toolbox with things to feel stronger. It's exciting to take a more active role in my healing by finding complementary treatments.

My Birthday
Monday, August 5, 2013, 12:25 p.m.

I was an only child and benefited from a fifteen-year generation gap between me and my cousins, so my birthday was always celebrated like a national holiday. We'd have a kid party and a grown-up party—and we'd prepare both for weeks in advance. I was showered with gifts and was the center of attention. Along with a cake (always made by my grandma), root-beer floats were often part of the fun. The way the ice cream and carbonation bubble up to make a creamy foam makes pouring the float almost as fun as drinking it.

By the time I was in my twenties, birthdays seemed pretty dull by comparison, and by my thirties, I just wanted to forget about them. Now, given all that has transpired in the last few years, I feel so lucky to be having a birthday at all.

The best birthday gifts are intangible. A husband who loves me despite my many imperfections. A healthy, smart, talented, beautiful daughter who likes to spend time with me and will unload the dishwasher without moaning and crying—my wish for this year is that she'll start to load it eventually, but for now, touching a dirty dish is, in her words, "way too gross." Another favorite gift is a healthy, smart, talented, handsome son who constantly makes Lego creatures, cracks funny jokes, and finds cool rocks for me—and who gave me sixteen dollars in cash for my birthday this morning. (Jackson thinks cash is the best gift ever.) There are many other gifts to count too. An extended family who has loved me in all my weirdness since day one. A neighborhood that, like a family, finds a way to support and help each other every day despite and because of our collective quirks. In-laws, coworkers, church members, and all those people who walk into our lives at just the right time. You're all important to my healing process, and there's no way to thank you enough.

I'm at the end of my fourth (fifth?) cycle of Xeloda, and the side effects require me to nap more often, move a little less (sore joints and feet), and carry Imodium in my purse just in case. Overall, the side effects are tolerable, and I hope my next blood work reveals that it's still effective. While it's hard to curse a medication that is keeping the cancer at bay, I did count my pills the other day, a ritual I do toward the end of each two-week cycle. Counting out how many pills remain is reassuring; it's like seeing the light at the end of the tunnel. Tomorrow morning, I'll take my last dose and then have a week off.

Compared to a year ago, there are so many things that I can do. I can walk two blocks and back without fear of falling. I can walk through about half of a big box store. I can do more than one thing on most days. I have the strength to hold my son. I have a baby Chihuahua who doesn't mind wearing cute outfits. We can feel secure staying in our house, even though money is tight. I know that I'm able to contribute to society despite no longer doing the professional work I did in the past.

Stayin' Alive

Monday, August 19, 2013, 10:32 p.m.

Since my last post, I've seen Dr. Anderson. My numbers are holding steady. He suggested probiotics, which have been working to get rid of the diarrhea. The day my diarrhea ended, though, Lupita Maria's started. A peanut that fell onto the floor is the main suspect. Back when she was a puppy, we gave her peanut butter, and it made her barf. The stray peanut she ate the other day confirms she has a peanut allergy. What is this world coming to when classrooms ban peanuts for allergic kids and now even puppies have peanut allergies? We had to put her on a bland diet for a week, place puppy pads all over the house, and constantly clean up her squishy poo. Thank God we have hardwood floors.

In the midst of dealing with Lupie poo, we were getting ready for Vivian's first-ever surgery. She has an extra bone in her foot that makes wearing anything other than flip-flops painful. When the surgeon showed us the before-and-after X rays, she said that extra bone she removed was so big, we could have named it. We've known about the extra bone for years, but she wasn't a candidate for surgery until her feet stopped growing. Vivian was a little champion recovering. She still has three weeks on crutches and a knee scooter and then another month taking it easy in a medical boot. The timing was perfect in terms of shows, auditions, and school—she's at a lull with all of them. She'll miss soccer this year, but something had to give. Luckily, we've made our out-of-pocket maximum for the year, so this surgery was free.

Having Vivian and Lupie under the weather have both been blows to my mental health, evidenced by my daily crying. This is quite a feat for someone on antidepressants. Yesterday, I started crying in church and didn't stop for two hours. Not silent, Victorian-style tissue-dabbing crying but chest-heaving, primal-scream sobbing with tears exploding from my eyes. Yes, I appeared totally crazy. Most of the time, I wear my crazy with pride, but yesterday, not so much. At church, poor Jackson had to go up to Communion alone because I was paralyzed (this is before the really bad crying started).

A friend asked what depression feels like. For me, it's a sense of total hopelessness. It's needing to do a task like opening my e-mail and feeling totally overwhelmed at even just the thought. It's being in pain and seeing no way out of it. It's the feeling that one little negative vibe like a swear word cuts into what's left of my soul. It's a feeling that every choice I've ever made has been wrong. It's the sense that there are people in the world whose biggest worry is packing or unpacking for a vacation or the quality of the greens in their restaurant salad or the quality of the greens at their golf course. It's believing there are lucky people in the world, and I have never been, and will never be, a lucky person. It's the feeling that I've failed my family and they would be better off without me because I'm just a burden to them. I've been feeling quite active and useful to my family the last few weeks, so feeling like a burden now means my depression is back.

All the same, when I got home from church, I decided to take my nightly dose of lorazepam early so I could get to sleep. I dramatically asked Wade to remove all the other pills from the bedroom because it would have been too tempting to swallow them all. I've never made a suicide attempt, nor do I imagine I ever will, but there are times when the option of suicide is so attractive it becomes fixed in my mind. The whole time I was falling asleep, I thought about the (very dull) scissors in the bedside drawer and tried to recall the location of the jugular—while I would never want to leave a bloody mess, it would be the most efficient way without pills. Then again, I wouldn't want to feel the pain of dull scissors in my neck. I know pills aren't mess-free, but still.

I must have some luck left because I was able to go to Sunday dinner at my cousins' house and tell them how terrible I've been feeling and get support from family. It's hard to admit feeling like a giant mess, but when you do, people are so kind and supportive.

Yes, it's dark to think about suicide, but sometimes the pain settles in, and when I haven't been sleeping well, it seems like suicide is the only escape. Other women might wish to run to a spa, but I want a full escape or if not a full escape, perhaps a trip to the hospital psych ward? Again, I've never attempted it, and today I'm feeling rational. The pills by my bedside will be there in the morning because I don't have an immediate need to escape. I'll watch something funny on TV, read a book, and play a game on my phone. Tomorrow, I'll meet with my priest and try to find out where God has gone. I know God is probably carrying me now, just like in the cheesy "Footprints" poem, but it sure doesn't feel like it. It feels more like God is gone, and I can't find him. My faith has worn thin. The day after tomorrow, I'll also meet with my psychiatrist and psychologist. Today, I called the drug company and discussed the possibility of the chemo doing this to me—personality changes, depression, and suicide are listed as side effects. They didn't think so but encouraged me to talk with my oncologist.

So by not committing suicide, I've had a successful day. Pretty low standards when success is defined by not offing oneself. Or maybe it's the highest standard of all—it's difficult to stay alive when feeling overwhelmed by every little thing.

In the next few weeks, I'll work with my medical professionals to unravel the web that has me feeling stuck. Just for today, I have hope that we'll find solutions to make life more manageable.

How crazy to endure painful side effects and allow hundreds of thousands of dollars to be spent on my health care only to want it all to end because I can't handle what's left of my life.

Still Alive

Wednesday, August 21, 2013, 9:58 p.m.

I feel I owe you an update from my last journal. Yesterday, I talked with the pharmacy, Dr. Anderson, and my priest. The pharmacist insists my poor mood is not due to the chemo—and Dr. Anderson agrees. It's a relief because the chemo is working, and I don't want to quit it due to a side effect. Then my priest gave me good insight into the darkness that sometimes surrounds us.

I saw my psychiatrist and psychologist today. (It takes a village to keep me calm.) The psychiatrist upped my antidepressant dosage and is allowing me an extra lorazepam. When I told him I'd considered a trip to the hospital over the weekend, he asked what I expected to get from the psych ward. I explained that I just wanted some warm blankets and someone to bring me a turkey sandwich. In a word, comfort. That's what I'd experienced in the hospital after having my babies, and it was lovely. He explained the psych ward is more about making sure a person is safe, and there probably wouldn't be any warm blankets. Where can a girl go to get some snuggly comfort? I guess I'll have to wait until my next PET/CT scan; they always offer warm blankets. In the meantime, Lupita and the kitties, Cedric and Shu Shu, will have to suffice.

A Sobering Day
Monday, August 26, 2013, 9:05 p.m.

Today was a sobering day for many reasons.

This morning, I woke up feeling like I've been hit by a truck. Tomorrow is the last day of this Xeloda cycle. My entire body aches, mostly the joints. My whole trunk feels bruised, like I've been beaten up by the meds. I've been forgetting my probiotic pills for a few days in a row, so my gut is retaliating with explosive action.

Then, this afternoon, I attended my first funeral for a support group member, Karen. It was a lovely service. Along with two other support group friends, we met Karen's husband, daughter, mother, aunt, and uncle. We heard funny stories of her as a toddler. We saw photos of her before she had cancer. Her beloved red convertible with the top down was parked in front of the church—it was so perfect. In addition to photos, there were fun artifacts from her life—a trophy won by her purebred dog, her scuba tank painted with gumballs, a recent Halloween costume. Karen was a beautiful person inside and out. She had enough grace to fill an ocean. Everyone at the service felt ready to live out her legacy of kindness, grace, and truth. This is something her family explicitly asked that we all do, live her legacy. I feel more committed to making a positive difference in the world.

Saying good-bye to Karen is sad, but it's also terrifying. Eight short months ago, she was "fine," meaning her metastasis was "under control." Then a small sensation in her jaw sent her to the doctor, prompting a brain MRI, which discovered the cancer in her brain. She was still at her job until a month ago. The fast and steep decline was horrifying. Her ability to maintain dignity through the process was inspiring.

The other reason this is a sobering day is because twenty-seven years ago, sobriety finally stuck for me. Most everyone knows I don't drink, smoke, take (street) drugs, eat red meat or drink caffeine, I've written about that already. I'm practically a Mormon minus the special underpants. The reason is something I've shared with very few people.

At age twelve, I met alcohol. It was love at first taste. It happened at an amusement park, introduced to me by a girl a few years older and a million times cooler than I was. In her purse, she had snuck in some rum brilliantly disguised in little shampoo bottles. She generously shared with me. I continued to drink alcohol, any type, whenever I could find it. My mom only drank one glass of wine on holidays, so there was nothing around the house to steal, but there are a surprising number of sources where a teen can find booze. Over-the-counter diet pills included speed in those days, so they would always do in a pinch. Why Walgreens never questioned a ninety-five-pound girl buying diet pills, I'll never understand. By the time I was fifteen, I'd carefully researched harder drugs and determined my next poison. Not pot, because it made people lazy. Ecstasy was still legal, but I already had enough boys trying to paw all over me, so no thanks. Cocaine was something even the kids using it didn't recommend, because it's impossible to quit. So the careful research I did in my high school library (yes, I was a nerd even about drugs) led me to my perfect poison—LSD.

Just thinking about it all these years later, I remember how much I loved it, more than anything in the world. My love for it was almost like the love for a person. Except "Sid" was perfect, never disagreed with me, and consistently knew how to make my world a better place. My trips were few and far between, because acid is a drug that requires you to clear your schedule for a few days, but it was always worth the wait. In between, I'd take diet pills and drink alcohol when I could get it.

By sixteen, I was suicidal and desperately wanted to quit drinking and drugs. I tried AA, but it didn't work. So I put myself into an outpatient treatment clinic. Combined with AA, I graduated high school with almost a year of sobriety under my belt.

This was in the late eighties in the suburbs, so treatment wasn't a shameful thing. It was almost a rite of passage. Minnesota is the treatment capital of the world, after all. The first few days of treatment were difficult—they tear you down to build you up. Within a week, I found myself in the safest, most honest atmosphere I've experienced before or since. Going back to school was difficult because there everyone wasn't perfectly honest with their feelings all the time, and it was hard to get back to "normal" culture. My mom was supportive through the whole process but shocked to learn what I'd been up to when she was working long hours.

For years afterward, I attended AA meetings, internalizing the messages, reading *The Big Book* several times. The treatment center I attended believed in building a support network so one could eventually thrive without attending weekly AA meetings. This is different from other treatment approaches that encourage a lifetime of AA. After my five-year chip, I attended fewer meetings, relying on friends and family for support. Most know AA has twelve steps, but it also has twelve promises—and if you work the steps, you'll receive the promises. One promise is that "God will remove your desire to drink," and when that happened for me, I was able to resume a pretty "normal" life.

In the beginning, I told everyone why I didn't drink. It was an insurance policy for my fledgling sobriety. But then after the promise was fulfilled, I was able to simply say, "I decided at a young age drinking wasn't for me," or I'd just order a Shirley Temple and let people assume it's part of my quirky personality.

At the same time I quit drinking, I also turned away from meat, caffeine, artificial sweeteners, smoking cigarettes (which I tried, but I was allergic to smoke), and chewing tobacco (which I tried successfully, but it was just a fad). For a short time, I deleted refined sugar from my diet, but a girl needs one vice. I'd started working out at a gym before I got sober, so the whole notion of a "healthy lifestyle," including the gym, was something I really embraced until the metastasis proved to me that a healthy lifestyle doesn't always translate into a healthy life. Ugh.

Wade didn't know me when I was drinking, so he can't imagine me intoxicated. The closest he's been to seeing me drunk is when I'm falling asleep or waking up from surgery. I know there are times he wishes I would just chill out and drink a glass of wine. But for me, the stakes are too high. I found a better life without mood-altering chemicals and continue to believe that's the right choice for me. Twenty-seven years is a long time to solidify a habit, and even with nothing more to lose, I feel I'm living a better life experiencing all my emotions instead of attempting to drown them out with drink or drugs. Now that cancer gives me access to unlimited narcotics, I feel even stronger about sobriety. If my days are numbered, I don't want to miss a single moment. And to me, I would be missing out if I spent time intoxicated. While some sober people won't take any pain medication, I know that the dose I take is right to control the pain without controlling my mood.

For my first few years of sobriety, my "birthday" on August 26 would be celebrated with cards, cake, and dinner out. After about ten years, it became more of a reflective day of gratitude for me to remember that even when we've hit rock bottom, God is there. Then through the wisdom of a room filled with strangers, we can find healing. Now the strangers in my room aren't fighting for their lives against alcohol and drugs but fighting for their lives against cancer. It's all the same. It's strangers who within one hour become friends, confidants, sisters. It was so sad to say good-bye to one of those sisters today, but I know that like all the amazing people I've met through AA and cancer support groups, I'm better for having known her just as her presence made the world a better place.

A Sunny Day
Monday, September 9, 2013, 2:57 p.m.

Two weekends ago, we took a Saturday drive to Duluth as a family. Our nuclear family, plus most of my extended family. There were sixteen of us in all. The group included family from Minnesota, New Mexico, New York City, New York State, and Washington, DC.

The best way to describe our trip is a pilgrimage. We met for dinner in Duluth and then drove another hour north to Gooseberry Falls State Park. We went to remember my sweet, dear cousin Sunny, who died four years ago, on the day of my mastectomy. One of her favorite spots was Gooseberry Falls, and her family donated funds to have a bench installed so others could sit and enjoy her favorite place, as well. The spot Sunny's husband, Mike, and their kids, Kelsey and Alec, selected was breathtaking. It was made up of table-sized volcanic rocks—a lovely reddish color. Stunning pale turquoise lichen grew on the rocks. Between the rocks were tall prairie grass and trees. The spot juts out onto Lake Superior with a twenty-foot drop to the water. Looking down at the water from the edge, red-brown rocks cropped out of the water. The lake itself is dark blue with white waves crashing onto the rocks. It was a perfect sunny day, both literally and figuratively. The weather was just right for us to enjoy the view of the lake, sky, rocks, grass. All the colors reminded me of Sunny, the blue of her eyes and the reddish brown of her hair. Her family had chosen a perfect spot to remember her beauty.

We toasted with her favorite wine (us teetotalers used our phones to toast) and shared a few remembrances. Sunny's daughter, Kelsey, told us this was a place her mom said she could go to "fill her soul." We're a lively bunch, normally all talking at once. But after the toast, we settled into a holy silence. We sat on the bench, on the rocks, walked along the rocks and looked over the edge into the water. It's the first time I can remember sharing long minutes of quiet with my family. In that time and space, we were very much together in the silence. It was a lovely way to fill our souls, in a beautiful place on earth, remembering a beautiful woman.

Comfort without Carbs

Thursday, September 19, 2013, 9:12 a.m.

My scan was two days ago, and in a few hours, I'll meet with my oncologist to get the results. My "scanxiety" has been pretty moderate this time. More mindful eating is forcing me to deal with emotions directly instead of trying to bury them with carbs. Still, I've enjoyed a few bowls of breakfast cereal in the last two days as I await my appointment with Dr. Anderson. Last time I saw him, I binged on five mini cupcakes, cereal, and whatever else we had in the house the night before the appointment. Last night, instead of binging on carbs, I binged on new episodes of *Breaking Bad* that I've been saving for a rainy day. The stress of awaiting a doctor's appointment counts as a rainy day.

Today is Wade's birthday. Poor guy, it will be pretty dull for him. We go to the oncologist in a few hours, and then it's meet-the-teachers night at Vivian's school. We'll do gifts and cake in between, but we'll wait for Saturday night to get his birthday meal at his new favorite sushi place down the street.

Happy Scan!

Thursday, September 19, 2013, 6:08 p.m.

The news today was the best we could expect: no evidence of active malignancy. Hurray!!!! In my support group, we call it NED, short for no evidence of disease. This was the outcome I was expecting, since I've been feeling so good lately and I've had almost zero pain in my hips. The only reason I didn't mention this hopeful prediction earlier is I didn't want to jinx it.

The other good news is this—instead of going two weeks on Xeloda and one week off, I'll now start one week on, one week off. This should make the side effects even more manageable. It also means less Xeloda over time—instead of thirty-four weeks per year, it's only twenty-six weeks per year. I'll go back for blood tests in four weeks and a scan in another few months to make sure this lower dose is effective.

This result is so exciting! I feel better physically and emotionally, now that I have concrete evidence that the cancer is fast asleep. It's still there, but it's not active or growing. I can be at peace with it in my body knowing it's not doing any damage at the moment.

Sleepover Camp
Wednesday, October 2, 2013, 1:44 p.m.

Purifying ritual bath, Sufi dancing, listening to music with eyes closed, swimming in an infinity pool, drinking tea, putting words to feelings, articulating fears, fresh smoothies every afternoon, sitting by a poolside fire at dark, letting-go ceremony with words melting into water, a meditation walk through all the chakras, resting in a hammock in the woods. These are a few of the activities I did last week at an Infinite Boundaries Breast Cancer Recovery retreat. Specifically for women with metastatic breast cancer and facilitated by breast-cancer survivors, this was four days and three nights with my peeps. We learned so much from the retreat and from each other.

The experience felt like going away to a sleepover camp and making new instant friends. Unlike sleepover camp, we didn't have to rough it. In fact, it was the most luxurious place I've ever experienced, a spa in Wisconsin called Sundara. My private room had a fireplace, a sink made out of a beautiful ceramic bowl, a feather-top bed, windows that opened to the woods, and a shower with a dozen shower heads.

Spending four days away from family and the business of everyday life was beyond refreshing. I was able to connect with other women with metastatic breast cancer in deeply meaningful ways.

I felt the presence of my mom there in three different ways. When I first arrived, I was told the meeting room number—it was the same as my mom's house number. Then, the first night we ate dessert first, just like my mom loved to do. On the last day, as I walked a path alone, I locked eyes with a doe and her baby, reminding me of my mom and me, just the two of us. Feeling my mom's presence and the meaningful retreat activities combined into a transformative experience unlike any other. I'm so happy I took the time for a retreat.

A Model Life

Saturday, October 5, 2013, 10:36 a.m.

On Thursday night, Vivian and I got to be supermodels for Angels and Divas, a fashion show fund-raiser for the Angel Foundation. We had the royal treatment with hair and makeup by Juut Salon.

Vivian looked beautiful, and she had a blast with another twelve-year-old she met at the Angel Foundation's Kids Kamp this summer. Vivian's friend watches a lot of *Project Runway*, so she taught us and her own cancer-survivor mom how to rock it on the runway. We all had a blast. It was fun to get glammed up and pretend to be carefree supermodels for one night.

Weeds

Wednesday, October 16, 2013, 10:54 p.m.

Last week in the midst of my happy scan news, I was feeling like I could make plans for the future. We made some travel plans for the next few months and scheduled a pottery sale, and I arranged to do some activities with Vivian. It's the first time in ages that I've been willing to look three months ahead, and it's been great to feel like things are somewhat stable.

Then I found out a metastatic friend has been given a six-month prognosis. This news reminds me of the Buddhist principle that stable ground beneath our feet is an illusion. She has kids a bit older than mine, and she feels comfortable that her husband will do a good job with them when she's gone. But it's really terrifying to know someone else who was fine a few months ago and is now walking toward the end of her journey. Sometimes I can feel peaceful about death, but right now, it seems horrifying. It also makes me so angry that humankind hasn't figured out how to kill a few little cells. Microscopic cells. How hard can it be? We've invented a million different ways to kill each other, and we can't find an effective way to kill a few errant little cells? Give me a break.

Over the weekend, I was able to experience some peace preparing our garden for winter. I pulled leftover veggie greens, stirred the compost, and pulled weeds. As I did these things, I smelled the wonderful compost odor—it's the smell of fresh horse poop, and to an urban farmer, it smells wonderful, because I know it will mean even better veggies for next year's garden. As I pulled the weeds, I thought about how even the bad things in life become part of the life cycle. The weeds I pull now will compost and nourish our food next summer. I've also realized that those who come before us continue to live on in so many unexpected ways. Even the bad weeds can nourish us by showing us how not to live. And the wisdom of those who come before us will nourish us with the words we need to survive today and improve the future.

It was fun to feel hopeful about our summer garden even as we prepare for winter. If I'm around to see the fruits of my labor, that will be a bonus, but doing the work itself is worth it even if I personally don't benefit from it. I enjoy pulling weeds; it is always a relaxing and meditative exercise for me.

Speaking of weeds, everyone in our support group has been offered weed by friends—so now we're all privy to know who among our friends and families smokes the stuff. We also have open-ended prescriptions for potentially mood-altering painkillers. But what's surprising is that none of us want them. While some of the women I know have an occasional cocktail, none of us want to misplace our consciousness, even for a short time. We realize how precious the present moment is, so we want to remain present in it. Most of us do take antidepressants and antianxiety medications, but those don't alter mood so much as increase resiliency. In other words, they keep us from spending our days crying.

Vivian's school conference was today, and none of her teachers had a bad thing to say about that little stinker. She's getting all As, so we celebrated, just the two of us, with lunch at her favorite restaurant. She's such a good little kitten. I'm so proud to say that I grew her in my tummy.

Feeling Better
Tuesday, October 29, 2013, 9:43 p.m.

Wade made me get out of bed and go to today's Day of the Dead celebration at the History Center. Jackson made a memorial box for our dearly departed dog, Savannah, and put it on her grave in the backyard when we got home. Vivian made one for my mom. It was a very colorful celebration, and I'm so glad we went.

Today was my last day of chemo pills for a week. The one-week-on, one-week-off schedule is wonderful. I just love it. I didn't even realize until tonight that it would be my last dose for a week. What a nice surprise!

Wade's working on some wonderful small-scale paintings, and we're both really excited to show them to everyone at his pottery and painting sale. We're also looking into getting them reproduced so he can sell signed prints at a lower price than the originals.

On Thursday, we'll have our tenth annual Halloweenie Roast. We can't believe we've been doing it for so many years! Wade sets up a table in the front yard, and the kids from our block and two other blocks come over for hot dogs and juice boxes before trick-or-treating. It's always so fun to see the kids in costume. The homemade ones are always the best costumes. Jackson wants me to revive my evil lunch lady from a few years ago, but I'm not sure what happened to the vital piece of the costume: the hairnet. I'll have to look for it.

Thanks to everyone for supporting me through all the ups and downs. Trying really hard to allow anger to inform me without letting it overtake me.

Chased by Nazis
Wednesday, October 30, 2013, 11:37 a.m.

Last night, Vivian had a difficult time getting to sleep because of a sore tummy. We stayed up and watched a few episodes of *Modern Family*, which made us laugh out loud. After that, she kept coming into my room and saying she couldn't sleep, and I kept kicking her out. She wouldn't take any medicine, and there wasn't anything she could say she needed. I should have snuggled the poor little thing and let her sleep in my bed, but I don't want to get sick from being close to her.

Then I had several dreams about living on a post-apocalyptic type of island with, oddly, a twenty-two-story housing building at the center. This was not a tropical island. It was a totally gross concrete island. Nazis showed up from time to time to sweep the building and shoot all the Jews. I knew my dark hair and tan skin meant I was screwed. The Nazis were dressed more like modern-day white supremacists, so they weren't as easy to identify as the old-timey swastika-wearing types. Totally stressful dream. I spent the whole time running or hiding by scrunching up inside of closets and lockers or under desks and tables. At one point, I got outside and into a car, but I kept seeing the Nazi cars. No matter what I tried, I couldn't escape. It wasn't just me they were after but a bunch of the people on the island. Some people they didn't bother. Some of the safe people, like the collaborators of World War II, were willing to help me hide.

As always, my dreams uncover my deepest fears. The Nazis must be the cancer cells, and I'm running as fast as I can and hiding as well as I can to save my life. In my dream, there was a secret floor at the very top of the building that I could access for some relative safety, but not total safety. I think this means that while my waking life is going pretty well, I still have so many fears around cancer. In my waking life, just one little twinge of pain in my hip sends me into a terrified state. I need to change my focus to all the positives that are outweighing the negatives at this moment. But I still have to acknowledge the fear and the real danger that the cancer can wake up at any time. Nazis suck. Cancer sucks.

Return of the Evil Lunch Lady

Friday, November 1, 2013, 1:09 p.m.

Per Jackson's request, I reprised my role as the evil lunch lady for Halloween this year. The wart on my chin was my own 3-D creation, made from those "boogers" that you get from coupon cards held on through the mail with glue. I colored the booger black with eyeliner and then added a tine from a hairbrush and glued it on with eyelash glue, creating the perfect hairy mole. Jackson said the facial hair and unibrow I created with mascara were the most disturbing parts of the costume.

I lacked a proper food-service hairnet, so I had to substitute an old-school grandma hairnet from the pharmacy at the last minute.

We had more kids than ever trick-or-treating. Almost all the hot dogs at our Halloweenie roast were gone before the night was over.

The Phoenicians

Thursday, November 21, 2013, 5:17 p.m.

A few weeks ago, Vivian, Jackson, and I attended my cousin Laura's wedding to John in Phoenix. The ability to pay for this expensive trip was provided by our generous friends and neighbors who surprised us in May with the party and "family memories fund."

The Phoenix wedding invitation arrived when I was still on my Dr. Anderson–induced summer travel ban, so I wasn't sure if we could attend. Then, after my last scan was so good, I decided to take the kids. I'm sorry that Wade had to stay home for work.

It was so fun to be with my cousins Jeanne, Monica, and Nancy and their families. The groom's dinner was at our hotel, outdoors with wonderful southwestern food and a classic mariachi band. At one point, I told the kids I was going up to our room and asked if anyone wanted to come with me to use the bathroom. The kids said no, but Jackson asked that I bring down a five-dollar bill from his travel bag. He had earned four five-dollar bills before our trip doing some housework. I brought down his money, and he tipped the mariachi players five dollars! It was the highlight of my night. I love that he loved the music and that he is such a generous little man.

The wedding itself was at the Phoenix Art Museum, a lovely venue. We had so much fun at the dinner afterward, but poor Jackson melted down before the dancing started. So we went back to the hotel early, which was fine since I was tired too. Vivian was cheerful and helpful during the entire trip. She's an excellent travel companion.

On our last day in Phoenix, a kid drove his dad's car into the water main outside the hotel, so the city had to shut off the water to the entire hotel. That evening, I showed the kids how to flush a toilet with pool water. They learned how a toilet works and that the water doesn't even need to be clean to get it flushed. An important life lesson, right?

The next morning, the hotel water was still out. I was disappointed to not have a shower and that the hotel kitchen was still closed due to the water outage. After packing, we happily left early for the airport, deciding to get some breakfast there.

We arrived at the Phoenix airport hungry. I insisted we get through security and find our gate before we stopped to eat. After the security line, we walked toward our gate. There were so many people, wall-to-wall people. And thanks to our showerless morning, we were literally part of the unwashed masses.

After finding our gate, we went to one of those icky little airport counter cafés. As we entered, a man walked out, and our eyes met. I couldn't make this up, so you know it's the truth when I tell you that I looked at him and asked, "Are you David Sedaris?"

In a soft voice, he said, "Yes." I gushed about him being my favorite living author. I even pointed at Vivian and said, "When this one was born, I didn't bring a Bible or childbirth book into the hospital with me, but I brought *Me Talk Pretty One Day* in case I needed a good laugh to get through the labor." He laughed gently at that. I asked if I could hug him, and he kindly declined by saying, "No, I don't hug." So I asked for a photo, to which he happily agreed. In the photo, you can see Jackson's hand wiping away the tears I was crying. Normally, I feel sorry for famous people and don't approach them, but I broke my rule for David. Out of respect, I kept the interaction short, and after the photo, I said, "Thank you so much. I don't want to delay you; have a good flight." And he left for his gate.

At this point, I burst into tears like a teenage girl who'd just met Elvis. My kids were asking why I was crying and asking who that man was. A few people in the café asked who he was, and I explained that they must read his books because he's hilarious. I've always thought it was so stupid when teenage girls cry when they meet a band like the Beatles, but now I understand. My tears were totally uncontrollable. They weren't tears of sadness or joy, rather a powerful emotional release. I felt like my life was complete.

My only regret with the photo was that because we had no water, I hadn't even bothered to even wash my face with bottled water, nor had I bothered to put on a stitch of makeup, so my face is plain in the photo, but I love the photo, anyway. David is only a few inches taller than I am, and he's just as adorable as I'd imagined.

Once I got my crying under control, reality set in when the café worker told me they were no longer serving breakfast and we'd have to choose salads or hamburgers for breakfast. But at that point, it didn't matter, I'd met my favorite author, and we were on our way home.

It was an exciting trip, and it only cost me one full day of sleep once we got home. My kids and I spent quality time with family and witnessed a lovely wedding. The kids learned some life skills, and I met my hero. I never did tell the kids—or David, for that matter—about my wonderful vacation last year during my MRI with David Sedaris.

Our Thespian Lifestyle
Monday, November 25, 2013, 10:30 a.m.

Soon after my initial diagnosis in 2007, Vivian found her passion in theater. She loves to see and perform in shows. Singing and acting are her favorite things, and she's also learned to love some aspects of stage management. She's a true thespian. And for a twelve-year-old, she has an impressive résumé.

The very first show she did was *The Best Christmas Pageant Ever.* At that first audition, they encouraged me to audition too, because they needed a few adults for the show. I'm a good sport, so I tried out, but when we were both called back, I took a careful look at the rehearsal schedule and realized it would be impossible to take that much time off work. I was already miles behind at the office from so much time off for surgeries and chemo.

Each year since that show, Vivian has asked if we could audition together again. Last year I was way too sick, but this year, when auditions for *The Best Christmas Pageant Ever* came around, I was feeling pretty good, so I tried out. Vivian scored the role of Maxine, the narrator of the pageant within the play. I got the role I was hoping for, Mrs. Edna McCarthy, a gossipy church lady.

The story is a heartwarming comedy that centers around a church Christmas pageant that is the same every time—until this year, when six naughty siblings, the Herdmans, decide to take over the roles of Mary, Joseph, the Wise Men, and the Angel of the Lord. Chaos ensues, and the church ladies have a field day gossiping about these rotten kids who shouldn't even be allowed into church. In the end, the Herdmans teach us that sometimes it's people from the fringes of society who can show us the true meaning of Christmas.

In addition to being gossipy, as Edna McCarthy, I get to do something illegal—I get to scream "Fire!" in a crowded theater. It's something I never thought I'd do! The last (and first) time I did a play was when I was seven and played the lion in *The Wizard of Oz.* It was really fun. I'm not sure why I waited thirty-five years to do another play. We've been in rehearsals for several weeks already, and I look forward to the performances. It's beautiful to see Vivian in her element.

Another Good Scan!

Monday, December 9, 2013, 10:08 p.m.

Got this morning's scan results earlier than normal—everything looks GOOD! The cancer is still there, but it's not active. It means the Xeloda is still working.

Vivian and I had five performances of our play over the weekend, with twenty-one more to go in the next two weeks. It's so much fun. The audience loves it, and everyone laughs a lot. I still have several places in the show where I have to stifle a laugh.

This show has tested my physical limits—I'm walking up and down many stairs and walking (sometimes at a slow trot) across the stage and lobby. This doesn't sound like much, but it has me thinking that once the show is over, I can start to add some real exercise to my daily activities.

New Year's Eve

Tuesday, December 31, 2013, 7:06 p.m.

There is so much to reflect upon from the past year. So many happy things have happened. The biggest one was finding a medication that works for me! The Xeloda is keeping the cancer from spreading and even killing some of the little monsters that have been lurking—all with manageable side effects.

Just one year ago, my mobility was quite limited. Now after doing the play with Vivian, I understand I'm capable of so much more physical activity than I've been able to do in years. This improvement in physical mobility gives me hope for the future.

Some of the year's other highlights: traveling; lovely holidays with the kids and family; my friend Karen's funeral (yes, a funeral can be a highlight); speaking at a few cancer charity fund-raisers; wild laughter and cleansing tears at my metastatic breast cancer support group; helping two students in Jackson's class learn to read; spending time with Vivian in her natural habitat, the theater; performing for developmentally disabled adults during the run of the play; late-night stops at SuperAmerica with

Vivian for doughnuts after rehearsal and then staying up late giggling, eating doughnuts, and watching TV; modeling with Vivian in the Angel Foundation fashion show; seeing Jackson learn things at the science museum and children's museum; watching him play with his Legos and laugh with his friends; and experiencing the extreme generosity of so many individuals helping our family as we continue to live with cancer.

Most importantly, I realized I can be fully alive today, making short-term plans for the future, understanding they can change at any time and being OK with it. That's all life can offer any of us. As the New Year waits on the horizon, I'm thankful for the ability to really live life one day at a time. Today, I'm centered in the now, relishing the gifts of this present moment.

afterword

I was nervous and naive as I anticipated my first chemo class in October 2007. I jokingly dubbed it Camp Chemo because I knew it would be a kind of medical boot camp to prepare me for the upcoming treatments. Humor helped me face the scary and mysterious process of chemo. I had no idea how much Camp Chemo and other unexpected cancer adventures would transform everything. If I'd known that cancer would become the compass to my everyday life—for the rest of my life—the newly diagnosed me would have been infuriated and terrified. In my early months with cancer, I was sure my Stage III diagnosis was just a speed bump.

The "camp" metaphor turned out to be more apt than I initially realized. Camp Chemo implies a kind of militaristic boot camp rife with constant distress and overwhelming fatigue. It's a place that breaks you down but eventually builds you back up again and endows you with a new purpose. I couldn't always choose my circumstances, but I learned I could sometimes choose my perceptions. Now, as I continue to navigate life with cancer, I often consider whether or not I've moved on to other kinds of camp.

Sometimes life feels like a sleepaway camp. Like a child forced to participate by well-meaning adults, I feel nervous, homesick, and far away from everything familiar. I'm making do with the limited resources on hand—and sometimes more than anything, I just want to be back in familiar territory. At other moments, I'm happy to be learning new skills and making new friends among my fellow campers, who are growing and changing as much as I am from a shared intense experience. I know that when I get back, my home will seem changed because I will return altered.

Sometimes life feels like a prison camp. I never signed up for this in the first place, and I'd rather be back at home instead of housed in a barracks of symptoms and forced into a parade of procedures. Stripped of wealth, relationships, abilities, and freedom, sometimes it seems the only way out is death. As my inner reserves are tested, eventually my barest, truest self is revealed. It feels possible that I'll never see home again.

Sometimes life with cancer feels—happily—like day camp. I'm here, we're all here, to learn something new. We are enriched, comforted, and made better by what we're learning with our fellow campers. But at the end of the day, we go back home to our families, back home to what's most familiar. We choose what we'll do with each day and the rest of our lives.

As I continue to navigate life with metastatic breast cancer, I ask myself, *Which camp am I in today?* Like it or not, cancer has become my compass, but I still get to decide in which direction it guides me. It's a metaphor that helps me remember what I learned reading Viktor Frankl's *Man's Search for Meaning* as a college freshman: We can't always choose what happens to us, but we can choose how we react.

I began writing CaringBridge blog entries as a practical way to communicate about my cancer diagnosis and treatment with my support network. Then, as the months and years passed, it transformed into reporting about life with cancer. Eventually, even while I was in the middle of a treatment or another cancer-connected incident, I'd be thinking about how to write about the experience for the blog. The entries were often composed in the car while I was driving home from work or medical appointments. By the time I'd get to the computer, it didn't take much time to put my day into words. The whole time, my supportive family, friends, coworkers, bosses, and neighbors were reading along. They encouraged me to share my writing more publicly, but I was so busy trying to keep my head above water that I didn't have time to make that happen. I only became motivated to publish my story for a wider audience after I discovered how misunderstood metastatic breast cancer is.

The current accepted breast cancer narrative in our culture is this: A diagnosis leads to surgery, chemo, and radiation, and then you're a survivor. However, in about 30 percent of people with breast cancer, the disease metastasizes. Doctors have no way to predict who will experience metastasis and who won't. The average life span for someone with metastatic breast cancer is only two years.

I hope this book will help people better understand metastatic breast cancer through a glimpse into one person's experience of it. I believe in the power of stories. I hope my story will inspire others to tell their stories, and together we'll shine the light of awareness on this largely hidden aspect of breast cancer. Only then will we end this disease.

Cancer changed my world dramatically, but I still have goals to accomplish and ideas to explore. I know my future plans will unfold slowly and not always according to schedule. But today is a good day. My pain level is minimal. My mobility is good. I'm well rested. A newly FDA-approved medication is keeping the cancer asleep. My husband and kids are healthy. Those are blessings to be celebrated.

Whatever the future holds, at this moment, I'm able to meet it with energy and pragmatic optimism. I wish the same for you.

Camille Scheel

July 7, 2015

The story continues at CampChemo.com.

Acknowledgements

To thank everyone who helped our family over the years would result in a tome the length of a phone book. Please know that I have appreciated you all. Here are a few shout-outs to some of the many people who helped with this book.

Everyone who read and commented on my CaringBridge posts. Your early feedback that my writing helped you motivated this book.

Peter Clowney, without you this project would not have happened. Your generosity, gentle guidance, extreme intelligence, and sharp editing made this book better. I treasure our conversations, and I cannot thank you enough.

Steve Nelson and Sarah Lemanczyk, for recommending Peter Clowney.

The folks at Beaver's Pond Press: Lily Coyle, for your belief in this project from day one, for your enthusiasm for the *Camp Chemo* title, and for making the arduous process of publishing fun; Wendy Weckwerth, for your careful and intelligent edits; Laura Drew, for your patience and for creating the beautiful book design; Kevin Cannon, for sticking with me as we hammered out the *Camp Chemo* logo; and Chris and Sara Ensey, for your sharp eyes and early praise for *Camp Chemo*.

Stephanie Gerster and DeAnn Dankowski, for your thoughtful comments. (I'm sorry that early manuscript was so long!)

Barb Gehlen, for being a dear friend and for reading both the CaringBridge blog as it was created and later the *Camp Chemo* manuscript.

Sister Marie Shaun, for reading my entire CaringBridge at once, all those years ago. You made me feel like a real author.

Joe Garbarino, for planting the seed to create a book from my CaringBridge, back before I ever thought it was possible.

Lynn Giguere, for the great author photo.

My Indiegogo backers for helping finalize the financing for this book: Kristin Muller, Clark Rexrode, Talia Camarena, Donald and Julie Morath, Richard and Sue Wynne, Nina Muller, Julia Ferguson, Gene Scheel, Stephanie Hansen, Heather Anfang, Penny Heaberlin, Marcy

Wengler, Jennifer Kinkead, Laura Bell, Holly Stoerker, and Melissa and Uri Camarena.

Doctors—those mentioned by pseudonym and those who aren't mentioned—your knowledge, love, and expertise saved my life.

The many nurses, whose love and care will always be remembered. You really are angels on earth.

Cancer researchers everywhere, your creativity and commitment gave me life enough to complete this book.

My lymphedema therapists, for remaining hopeful during my darkest times.

Mental health professionals, for teaching me coping strategies, even when I was feeling most out of control. Sandi Tazelaar, for your wisdom. Gayle Sherman Crandell and Katie Houselog, for thoughtfully co-facilitating a meaningful support group.

Social workers and teachers, for your expertise and heart: Cathie Duncan, Anna Garnaas, Lori Seastrand, Emily Madland, Sue Wynne, Maureen Burns, and so many more. You have my constant admiration.

And our amazing family:

Melissa and Uri, for caring so deeply about our kids. Your Sunday dinners became a lifeline for us to connect with family.

Mike and Ruth, for being my godparents and modeling how to live for the things that really matter.

Nina and Bob, for hosting me so often at your home and visiting us so often.

Kristin, you hold a special place in my heart as a kindred spirit and cherished friend. I love you, little cousin.

Kurt and Mary Kate, for staying in touch despite the miles that separate us.

Mike Forde, for attending Vivian's performances.

Alexa, for your kindness, for being there for Vivian, and for your medical advice as you became a doctor.

Talia, Kelsey, and Alec, for always staying in close touch with us even when you're far away.

Ron, Justin, Paul, Craig, and Izzy, for being lovely additions to our family.

Jeanne, Monica, and Nancy, for accepting me into the family and helping me understand who I am.

Mike and Stu, for being so welcoming.

Laura, for sharing photos of my father when he was young.

Nick, Dave, Justin, Katie, Patrick, and Ben, for being so kind and fun.

Gene and Beckie, for raising a great bunch of kids and for being caring grandparents.

Kent and Mary, for showing us the very definition of hospitality whenever we visit.

Mark and Barb, for caring about our kids and for the all-we-can-eat barbeque.

Carlene, for being one of my longest friends and for always talking so kindly about your little brother so that when I finally met him, I knew he was a good guy.

My neighbors, for your generosity and love: Deb and Ted, Lynn and Fred, Sara and David, Brenda and Steve, Naomi and Dave, Julie and Bob, Leslie and Michelle, Tom and Shannon, Trish and Ethan, JoAnn and Gary, Jennifer and Tu, Jean and Chris, Lori and Mike, Kate and Dave, Ray and Tori, Robin and Joel, Emily and Tony, Susan and Stan, Bill, Sheila, Karen, JoAnn, Maggie, Anne, and so many more. You make daily life delightful.

Minnesota Public Radio peeps, you are way too many to mention. Thank you for your daily conversation, for your ongoing concern, and for enduring my early attempts to voice my experience on stage.

My book group, for helping me become a more discerning reader and for all the laughter: Laura Bednarski, Judy Randall, Heather Anfang, Lisa Pugh, Sara Gross Methner, Colleen Eberhart, and Christine Esckilsen.

The congregation of St. John the Evangelist Episcopal Church for your prayers: The Reverend Barbara Mraz, for the thoughtful sermons; The Reverend Jered Weber-Johnson, for caring about our family from day one; The Reverend Frank Wilson, for your counsel during our darkest times; Jean Hansen, for suggesting and organizing a Healing Circle; Jennifer Kinkead, Jennifer Frost Rosendale, Kathy Brown, and Julia Ferguson, for reading, praying, and sharing your lives; Holly Stoerker, for helping me to see the hope in new friendship and for reading a draft of *Camp Chemo*; Dusty Mairs, for your enthusiasm and support for this project; Aimee Baxter, for your friendship and honesty and for your help with my author photo; Anneke and Andrew, Alice and Todd, Jennifer and Peter, Aimee and Tom, Laura Dale and John, for your friendship and carpools.

Shelly Palashewski, for sharing your love, wisdom, faith, and cabin. You are my longest friend. Thank goodness you laughed at my turtleneck joke way back in eighth grade!

Alison, for being the one I called as I drove to that first ultrasound, and for your generosity throughout this journey.

Angela, for keeping me in giggles over the years.

Dave and Irene, for Hotel Peterson and so much more.

Dan Kensinger, for your constant friendship and impeccable hospitality.

The Deneen family, for your friendship and generosity.

Laura Whitley, for being Lupita's home away from home and for being the very first one to send a note once news broke of my metastasis.

Stephanie Hansen, for following my story and generously sharing yours.

Kerry Durkin, for the cross-disease chats over tea.

Tina, Paul, John, and Melissa, for sharing Alice with us and for accepting Vivian as one of your own.

The women after my own heart: Deb Rae, Stephanie Gerster, Susan Rhea, Megan Schaefbauer, Penny Heaberlin, Christine Dwight, Lynn Sax, Kahron Palet, Sue Dwyer, and so many others. I love you!

Facebook meta-sisters, becoming a part of your community provides more support and laughs than I ever could have imagined.

The lovely women I met at Living Beyond Breast Cancer's Annual Conference for Women Living with Metastatic Breast Cancer in Philadelphia.

The congregation of St. Luke's Episcopal Church, for your continuing prayers.

St. Thomas More and J. J. Hill Montessori moms, faculty, and staff, for coming to the rescue so many times.

Everyone who sent a card, gift card, bag of groceries, or hot dish and everyone who organized meals, laundry, cleaning, childcare, and carpools. You've made our world a happier place.

For the organizations working to cure and support people with cancer, including CaringBridge, Living Beyond Breast Cancer, Metastatic Breast Cancer Network, Virginia Piper Cancer Institute's Piper Breast Center, METAvivor, Breast Cancer Education Association, Minnesota Breast Cancer Coalition, Gilda's Club of the Twin Cities and the Cancer Support Community, American Cancer Society, Susan G. Komen Race for the Cure, and the Angel Foundation, especially Margie, Janice, and Missy.

Wade, for starting this book with the very first post on my CaringBridge site and for being my rock to lean upon.

Vivian, for keeping me centered in the excitement and activity of everyday living and learning.

Jackson, for helping me laugh and experience joy even when I thought it was impossible.

Animal Humane Society of Minnesota, for providing the pets mentioned in this book.

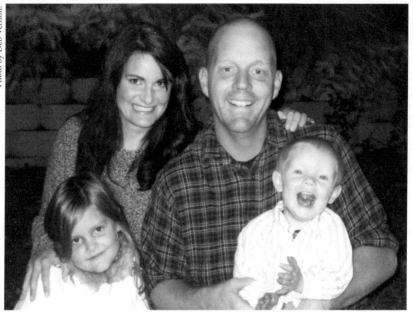

My family 2007

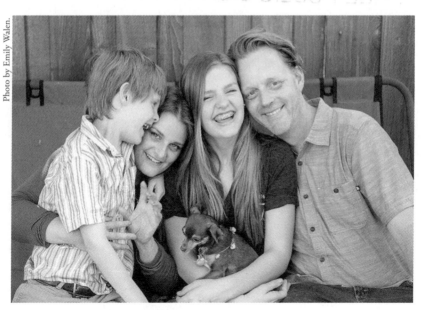

My family 2014